TELL ME
A SECRET

TELL ME A SECRET

TRUE CONFESSIONS OF BRITAIN'S MOST BEAUTIFUL EROTIC DANCERS AND MODELS

DAWN SIMPSON
www.dawnsimpson.com

JOHN BLAKE

Published by John Blake Publishing Ltd,
3, Bramber Court, 2 Bramber Road,
London W14 9PB, England

www.blake.co.uk

First published in hardback in 2005

ISBN 1 84454 120 7

All rights reserved. No part of this publication may be reproduced,
stored in a retrieval system, or in any form or by any means, without the
prior permission in writing of the publisher, nor be otherwise circulated
in any form of binding or cover other than that in which it is published
and without a similar condition including this condition being imposed
on the subsequent publisher.

British Library Cataloguing-in-Publication Data:

A catalogue record for this book is available from the British Library.

Design by www.envydesign.co.uk

Printed in Great Britain by CPD

1 3 5 7 9 10 8 6 4 2

© Text copyright Dawn Simpson 2005

Papers used by John Blake Publishing are natural, recyclable products
made from wood grown in sustainable forests. The manufacturing processes
conform to the environmental regulations of the country of origin.

In loving memory of my mum, Nancy, and my son,
Leslie – forever loved and never forgotten.

FOREWORD

Hi my name is Peter Stringfellow. I own the most prestigious tableside dancing clubs in the UK and one in Paris. The girls that dance there are beautiful. People travel for miles around to visit the Club, which naturally attracts the rich and famous.

I first brought tabledancing to London and the UK in 1996. Up until then Stringfellows had been an internationally famous Restaurant/Discotheque but since then my concept of beautiful girls dancing topless on stage and nude tableside has become such a huge success that Stringfellows is now synonymous with this form of entertainment. The success of the club is not just because the girls are drop dead gorgeous, but because of the service and the way the club is run. I think the more tasteful the presentation the more appealing it is.

Most people say that, because I am surrounded by these beautiful girls, I am the luckiest man in the world. Maybe I am. But you know it is all about respect. If you respect the girls and take time to get to know them and take an interest in them, I believe the girls will respect me also. It may sound a little bit chauvinistic, but in my book it isn't. It all stems back from my childhood. I attended an all boys school, and had no sisters, so girls were kept at a distance and naturally I put these girls up on a pedestal and still do to this day. So, yes, I guess I am lucky.

I agreed to do the foreword for this book because I believe that it is good to surround yourself with beautiful things, but equally I think it is better to understand the beauty within. This book discovers what lies beneath the gorgeous women who fill the clubs and magazines which fascinate and captivate us so much. It is a testament to the strength and respectability of the girls who work so hard in an environment that, although sexy and glamorous, is also fiercely competitive. It takes a special character to flourish in the world of glamour. This book is full of such girls.

Peter Stringfellow

ACKNOWLEDGEMENTS

Firstly I would like to thank my husband, Chris, and children, Kelly and Christopher, for their support and encouragement while I have been working on this book. Also to Lynn Bell, who has been my mentor in life – she has always believed in me. To my friend Jimmy, who gave me the opportunity to do this book. Photographer, James Tiger, and his crew Kerry Potter MUA/Lighting Asst, Jason Lane Camera/Lighting Asst, Adam Corbet Camera/Lighting Asst, and Tamsin who was make-up artist (MUA) for the northern shoots. Chris Dobson, Hotel Manager, of the Thistle Kensington Gardens, London, where most of the photography took place (he is also my little brother). I would like to thank Judy Broadbent from Custom PR for her support with the book launch. Last but not least to all the models and lap dancers in this book who shared their innermost secrets with me.

CONTENTS

Introduction ... xiii

NIKITA ... 1

TORI ... 25

DANNII ... 41

KAT ... 57

JESSIKA ... 79

ALEXANDRA ... 95

ELLIE ... 113

KACIE LOU ... 131

EMMA LOUISE ... 149

 FILIZ ... 171

 LUCKY ... 187

 FENYA ... 201

 HOLLYBLUE ... 213

 CHARLIE STORM ... 225

 DANI ... 259

 MADISON ... 271

 SARAH LOU ... 283

 NADINE ... 297

 KERRI D ... 313

 STACEY ... 337

 ZOE DEE ... 355

 YVETTE ... 377

INTRODUCTION

The sex industry is one of the largest in the world, and is worth billions of pounds each year. Sex, whether in the form of DVDs, magazines, or the entertainment on offer in lap-dancing clubs, has never been so popular, nor sold so well. Quite simply, the sex business holds a huge fascination for millions of us, whether we like to admit it or not! We spend our money on these things, and one look at the newspaper and magazine racks in your newsagent is evidence enough that we want to know all we can about the sex lives of the rich and famous. In an age where sex is no longer a taboo, men and women can celebrate and explore their sexuality in any way they choose. We all love sex, and we're more ready to admit it than ever.

One of the biggest growth areas, apart from online sectors, has been men's magazines, or 'lad mags', as we call them. In recent years, more and more of these 'middle shelf' magazines have hit the shelves. However different and unique the magazines try to be in order to compete in this aggressive market, regardless of whether they focus on men's health, sport or fashion, they all have one thing in common – gorgeous women, and lots of them! Glamorous, seductive girls fill their pages with their irresistible looks – sex sells, after all, and at the moment it seems we can't get enough of it.

The lad mag phenomenon has opened up all kinds of opportunities for girls to get into the glamour industry. Once upon a time, if a girl announced her career as a glamour model or lap dancer, she would have been shunned as if she has declared herself a prostitute. Now a career in glamour modelling or lapdancing is much more accepted, particularly by celebrities. Women can display their bodies for the pleasure of others without being made to feel cheap or dirty, and we too can enjoy what's on offer without it being a guilty pleasure.

Glamour models and lap dancers play a large part in the sex industry. They are the girls that satisfy our large appetite for sexy stories, they are the subject of many sexual fantasies, and very often a hot source of celebrity gossip. Think of how many models have sold a 'kiss and tell' story

INTRODUCTION

to the press, and on the back of it become rich, famous or both.

But what about the girls themselves? Do we ever stop to think who they really are? Probably not. Until I started to research and interview girls in this profession, I, like many others, had preconceived ideas of who they were. I assumed they were wannabes, choosing an easy career, 'all tits and no brains'. After all, what does it take to get your tits out for an hour and do a few sexy poses for a photographer? Get dressed, pick up a cheque – thank you very much. Or to do a three minute strip for some guy for £20? Not a bad hourly rate!

After the recent 'Jordan phenomenon' – Britain's No 1 glamour model with no make-up, appearing vulnerable and stuck in the jungle on *I'm A Celebrity Get Me Out Of Here*, enabling the public to discover the personality beyond the common portrayal of her as merely a glamour model, or eye candy – I was intrigued. Was Jordan a one off? I couldn't accept that she was the only model who seemed to be able to grow in popularity because of her personality, as opposed to what size her boobs were, or what celebrity she was sleeping with. Although we all bought her book to find out anyway!

It was at this point I decided to research the

industry and the girls that worked within it. In order to gain a full understanding of who these girls were, I decided to carry out interviews in all parts of the Country and at all levels of experience, in both the glamour and lap dancing industries. I needed to know if my cynical view of 'all tits, no brains' was true.

Meeting these girls was truly interesting. I had imagined that they would all turn up looking like they had just dropped off page three! In fact, they were all dressed down, not wearing much make-up, and looking almost 'normal' – not what I expected at all. 'It's just a job,' they all told me. I hadn't thought of it as just a job, but I suppose if you were in the Police force, you wouldn't go and socialise in uniform. Their make-up, false hair, nails and 10-inch shoes were just a uniform to them. Those who had a boob job classed it as an investment, just like getting an upgrade on a PC; it helped them to increase their earnings.

I discovered very early on that each of these girls was completely individual – they were all intelligent, interesting and unique. However, the thing that fascinated me most is that they all had a different story to tell. As the girls started to trust me, they began to tell me things that they had never told anyone before. Of course there were the sexy stories and celebrity encounters, but

INTRODUCTION

there were also a lot of life issues these girls had battled through. There was far more to these girls than met the eye. I had been proven wrong.

This was probably the toughest industry I have every encountered. One that only the strongest of individuals can survive and succeed in. They are all constantly on an emotional roller coaster. For every job, there are two hundred willing-and-able models. It's not just about your look; it's how determined you are and how hard you work at it. I remember one girl telling me about a casting she went for. It took her three hours to get there, over £100 in travel expenses, all for ten seconds of 'Thanks for coming, but sorry you are not what we are looking for'. How many of us would stand for that? Does this mean that the only way these girls get the fame they desire is to go down the route of selling their sexual encounters with celebrities to the Nationals? After all, it has worked for so many…

The glamour industry is such a complex industry, and it now fascinates me more than ever. I have an unbelievable amount of respect for these girls. Through my journey of discovery I have made some good friends. They have trusted me, and shared their most inner secrets. Listening to their stories has taken me through every emotion. I have laughed at the things they get up to, been shocked at some of their sexual encounters, and cried at some of the things they have been through in life. But, most of all, I have come away with the feeling of respect for every single one of them.

Now every time I open a magazine, newspaper or visit a lap-dancing club, I look past the aesthetic of these beautiful girls, and look at them in admiration. I always wonder who they are, but more importantly I always ask myself one question ...

'What are their *secrets*?'

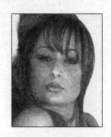

NIKITA

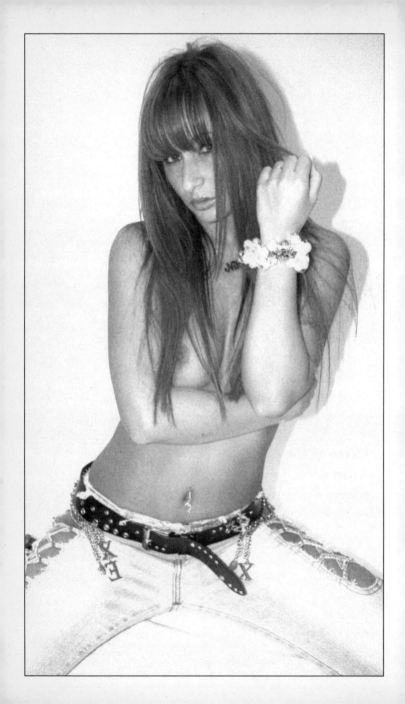

NIKITA

Name: Nikita Vassilliou
Model/Dance Name: Nikita
Star Sign: Cancer
Age: Model age 21 – real age 24
Vital Stats: 34B-24-three 4
Lives: London
Fave Food: My mum's cooking
Fave Drink: Water – it's Mother Nature's juice

Where do you work?

Apart from being a model, I am also a singer, rapper, songwriter, extremely small-part actress – oh, and I breathe fire as well.

I've been *Max Power* magazine's official promo babe for 2004, which involved me travelling all across the country and Ireland, promoting car shows. The work mainly consists of having my picture taken with fans and generally promoting the magazine.

TELL ME A SECRET

Last year I had the chance to prove that I'm more than a mannequin, as I was given the opportunity to perform my self-written track in front of over 10,000 people at *Max Power* Live in London. It was a great feeling, not only performing to a crowd, but the opportunity to be taken seriously – OK, the track was called 'Hot and Sticky' and involved lyrics such as 'Oh bend me over, baby, and give me some sucky licky', but, still, it was serious stuff for me!

I also recently learned to breathe and juggle fire and I am proud to announce that I still have my eyebrows, although I did burn my bum when my partner spanked me with my fire baton while it was lit!

I mentioned earlier about my 'small-part acting'. Well, to date I have managed to blag my way into a few films, such as Jude Law's *Closer*. I sneaked to the front of the set and managed to get a scene of me crossing the road with him! He was a bit stuck up towards me, even though I did the crossing the road scene for a good hour or so. When it rained, some bird came and held an umbrella over his lovely floppy hair, which I thought was a bit sad.

I also worked on the new *Charlie and the Chocolate Factory* starring Johnny Depp. No chance of meeting him though – I had to play a nut factory worker – oh, the glamour!

NIKITA

Other 'glamorous' jobs (apart from the time I was an intensive-care patient in *Holby City*) include fun things such as test driving a BMW Z4 for ITV. I had to stunt drive and was really enjoying it until the police pulled me over.

I've been in *Mile High*, *Footballers Wives* and appeared in newspapers such as the *Sport* – I like the *Sport* because they pay really well for minimum work! I was on Soccer AM for a few weeks, in which I had to have a bitch fight with a man dressed as a woman. My most recent job was playing a lap dancer in *Dream Team* – so I guess you could say I'm a bit of an all-rounder!

How did you get into modelling?

At the age of 21 I was jumping from job to job and couldn't really see any future in anything I was doing so, one day, I decided to do something about it. I needed to push my career in a direction that would keep me on my toes. I'm also a bit of an exhibitionist, so I sent copious amounts of cheesy underwear pics to many agencies and magazine competitions. I couldn't believe it when *FHM* told me I had got into the second round of Bikini Heaven. For the next round I had to re-make a scene from my favourite movie in just a bikini. When I think back now it was sooooo embarrassing. I wore an American-flag Wonder

Woman-style bikini and had masses of big blonde hair. I'd padded my boobs out to look like a couple of footballs. I know that the video is gonna come back to haunt me, but there you have it – my friend dressed as the killer and my boyfriend dressed as a woman, filming a scene from *Scary Movie*. We filmed it in my house and had scary sound effects playing on the record player. It was so funny – while 'the killer' was chasing me, you could see this record going round and round in the background making hideous groaning noises. I never made the third round – although I received a nice email from the editor saying it was the funniest thing he had seen in ages.

Even though I didn't get through, it got me interested in the modelling industry and I wanted more. I entered *Max Power* Star Babe and made the final 10. Because of this success, it gave me some ammo to go to the agencies with. A couple of them took me under their wing on condition that I lost two inches round my waist, grew back my pencil eyebrows, toned down the bleach-blonde hair, stopped lying about my bra size and started lying about my age!

Most of my work I negotiate independently from contacts I meet along the way, but one agent that helped me at the beginning was Sugarbabes. They sorted my first-ever portfolio pics out for

NIKITA

me with Andy Lesauvage. I remember I was so nervous as I'd always promised my parents and myself that I'd never go topless. The nerves lasted all of about 10 minutes.

It was funny when I first met Andy Lesauvage for my shoot. He marched straight up to my gorgeous friend, Debbie, who accompanied me there and said, 'Hi Nikita' and shook her hand. Well, I hadn't been made up and my hair wasn't done so I suppose I could forgive him that.

My second shoot was for Ben Westwood – Vivienne Westwood's son. Ben is as mad as a hatter, but is a great guy and takes the most unbelievable fetish pictures of me. That was my first encounter with rubber! It took me an hour to get the outfit on – I felt like a giant dildo! As well as a total twat posing in his kitchen sink. But the photos were so cool and kinda shocking at the same time. I sent them to London radio station Kiss 100's Bam Bam Breakfast Show. They invited me down to the studio, which resulted in me doing regular stunts out and about with 'Streetboy', the shows main entertainer. The stunts include things such as bikini car-wash wars etc. We both stood at 8am washing windscreens in bikinis for all the London rush-hour traffic. It was so funny. Another time, 'Streetboy' and I moonied on the Piccadilly Circus Eros Statue. We had to run from the police who were going to arrest us for indecent exposure.

Well, that was the early days. I still shoot with Ben Westwood, although I'm not so scared of rubber these days!

What's the biggest fee/tip you have ever earned?

I worked as a Performance Bikes Grid Girl at the Superbike Championships in 2004 and was paid £100 every time I opened the umbrella for a race. It was only opened for three minutes at a time. And then closed again. I sat around for the rest of the day sunbathing till the next race. They even paid my travel home. I know it's not extortionate but, still, that's big bucks for me. I can't believe I am admitting this but I once got paid £100 to smoke four ciggies for a cigarette-fetish guy. I even made him buy my cigarettes. I was desperate for the cash.

What highstreet publications have you been in? Have you worked with any famous people?

OK – once I did a mock-up paparazzi shoot and sold it to the *Sport*. The paper said I'd been sunning it up in my villa in France – when, in actual fact, I was really freezing my tits off in Loughton! I've also done Page 3 for them shot by Jeff Kaine. He is one top guy and I have a lot of respect for him.

I've worked with Lucy Pinder and Michelle

Marsh, who are really famous models at the 'Need For Speed 2' launch at the Ace Café. I was really nervous but they were really friendly and made me feel very comfortable. Unlike Jordan – she was less friendly when I first met her backstage at the *Max Power* Live 2002 show. I found this really disappointing, because I have always had a lot of respect and looked up to her.

Garry Bushell, however, is lovely. I did my first ever newspaper interview for the *Sunday People* and he was really friendly and easy to chat to. I worked with Tim Lovejoy on Soccer AM, although I didn't work on it this season, because a member of his film crew kept sending me naked pics of himself and I threatened to go to the papers – sad git. I also worked with Tim Westwood (radio one DJ and friend of Eminem) at Max London but we had a big argument and I still have not forgiven him!

When I played a lap dancer, I danced for one of the main stars in *Dream Team* in the new series. I was pretty useless on the pole – I slide down it like Fireman Sam, which is not a very flattering image!

I have worked with some well-known actors through my acting, including Jude Law, Gary Oldman, Joseph Fiennes, Heather Graham and Natalie Portman. Oh, and Tim Burton directed me in *Charlie and the Chocolate Factory*.

TELL ME A SECRET

What other work have you done?

I was an obnoxious kid – moody, pale and stick-thin. I looked like a boy and never had a boyfriend. Boys used to pick on me. I wasn't popular and was crap at sports. In fact I was a terrible truant! However, I did concentrate in lessons such as English and art – I surprisingly ended up with nine GCSE's, five of which were A and A*. I also managed to earn myself two A levels. But after that I jumped from job to job. I hate authority and got bored easily. That's why I love modelling so much. I do something different every time. There is no time to get bored.

Previous 'career' moves have been receptionist, credit controller, telephone sales, sales team supervisor, insurance sales, insurance claim handler, recruitment consultant, asbestos removal sales etc etc. I always quite enjoyed sales. I think that's because I love a good blag!

I'm now a self-employed model. But when I'm not taking my clothes off, my old boss, Terry, lets me come in and work for my old company, Universal, selling voice and data equipment. It's quite an involved job and you have to speak to some really interesting people. If I weren't modelling I would have liked to retire there. They have been very kind and supportive of my career.

NIKITA

Who knows, when my tits sag to my knees I may go back there and work full-time!

Do you have any famous friends?
Not really. I do stay away from the pretentious London celeb clubbing scene. I've got lots of friends in and around Enfield and Herts, but none is really famous. But my dad went to school with Jazzy B from Soul to Soul; my mum used to do Super Gran's hair and my auntie went to school with the two women off Birds Of Feather.

Mike McClean (some dodgy TV presenter) asked me on a date though – I laughed as he is just so cheesy. Why can't Robbie Williams ask me on a date, for goodness sake?

What does your family think of the work you do?
Half of them don't know what I really do. My dad is Greek and was quite strict when I was a kid. Telling him that I was going topless for the *Sport* was hard, but he said, 'Whatever makes you happy.' My parents know deep down that I am not naïve and that I won't do anything I feel uncomfortable with. My mum probably guessed I'd get into modelling. She is very attractive and still looks quite young. I think, if she hadn't married young and settled down, she could have been a really good model herself.

My nan, bless her ... she loves it. She was telling the ambulance men a few months ago that her granddaughter is a model. She then got out all my photos and said, 'Oh she definitely gets her looks from me'!

To be honest, some members of my family are proud of me, like my fiancée, Rob, my sister, Sam, who's 20, and my brother, John, who's 12 – I have a lot of time for them and will look after them when I really start to reap the benefits. Those that are against my chosen career path can kiss my ass, family or not. At the end of the day, it's my life and no one is going to stand in the way of my ambitions.

What's your funniest moment?
This is funny but embarrassing ... When I was about 14, I used to think I was really cool and hang out with lots of boys. One night we were all sitting on the fence outside my house in Cherry Road, Enfield. I can't remember what I was doing, but I was showing off as usual, because there was a boy in the group I really fancied. I was showing them how toned and trim my stomach was. I asked one of them to 'test the firmness' of my abdominal muscles. With that he punched me hard in the stomach and I let out this almighty rip of a fart in front of all the boys.

NIKITA

Those poor shocked boys. No one laughed. They were just stunned that something that loud could come from a girl. I ran to my house and didn't come back out for about three weeks. I'd have left the country given the choice!

Although my personal best funny moment was when I was going out with an ex-ex-ex-yummy. He was a half-Maltese Thai boxer with black hair and green eyes. He asked me to bring a girlfriend out one night to pair up with his mate for a blind date. I took along a right slapper who lived on my estate who would basically shag anything. I knew she would be a sure thing and I'd get to be alone with my man after all.

I was right. We met in Taylor's Wine Bar and after an hour of Jack Daniels and Coke she was anyone's. She went home with this other guy, who failed to tell her he still lived with his dad. That was the end of that, or so I thought. His mate rings the next morning going berserk. Basically he'd took my easy friend home and shagged her. She went to the bathroom, still completely pissed, then she staggers back into bed.

At 7am, this bloke's dad gets up for work and sees this very naked blonde bird in bed with him. Bearing in mind they must have been in bed asleep TOGETHER for about six hours (I swear to you this happened), he wakes her up shouting,

'Who the f*** are you?' She wakes up screaming, 'Who the f*** are you?', thinking she's gone home with a balding, middle-aged, hairy-backed slob in her drunken stupor.

The guy she really did do it with has woken up by now and rushed through into the bedroom, to catch his evening's conquest in bed with his dad. The pair of them were naked in bed repeatedly trying to convince the son that nothing happened, saying, 'it's not what you think!'

I swear it happened. It was 1997 and I'm not using my friend as a disguise for myself!

What's your scariest moment?

I didn't even need to pause to remember this one. Again it was 1997 and I was smoking illegal drugs with my friends – three boys and one girl. We were in a little Renault Clio parked in Epping Forest at 1am. We were parked in a ditch with the lights off. There was a church opposite and I could see these two people with painted white faces walk to the church and stand outside. Like they were keeping watch or something. I'm such a scaredy cat, plus I was stoned and paranoid, so I said to my mates, 'Please can we leave?' Boys will be boys and they were acting all macho: 'Don't worry, there's only two of them, we will protect you, baby'. We sat through another 15 minutes or so of me screaming like a baby that I wanted to go home. I was scared. Finally the driver of the Renault goes to me, 'Fine! I'll scare them off then' and he starts flashing his lights and sounding his horn like a lunatic. Well, that was clever. We looked to our left and there were about another 60 or so of these white-faced people walking up the road, swinging on the trees and sitting on the gravestones in the church. I don't know what they were doing there but we didn't stick around to find out as they all charged at the Clio. We managed to wheel-spin our way out of that ditch before we were all sacrificed!

My adrenaline is going mad now just thinking about it!

Have you ever turned down work and why?
I went to a casting and I got the job! It was to play strip poker on this programme on *Men and Motors*. I thought, Cool, I'm a dab hand at poker so the others will never get me naked. I turned up for the dress rehearsal. It was so tacky and the game was obviously fixed. I just walked out. I'm glad I did. I spoke to a mate of mine who took part and apparently it still gets repeated and can do for up to three years.

I also turned down a shoot for a website called Chicks in Diapers ... ooooh I wonder why?!

And I turned down a part in a Gary Oldman

film called *Dead Fish*. I was going to be a topless waitress. That wasn't the reason why I turned it down. When I got there my dad had been booked as an extra on the same film. I was gutted as it was paying really well. But I didn't want my dad to give up his part and I certainly wasn't going to walk around with tassels on my tits in front of him!

Do you have a sexual fantasy?
I have a quiet birthday gathering, which goes well. At the end of the day there are just a few of my celeb lad mates left. This is when the fun starts. First of all Robbie Williams starts snogging me. At the same time Freddie Ljungberg then goes down on me, pushing my Janet Reger pearl-gusset French knickers aside. Charlie from Busted and Lemar sing to me, while Johnny Depp films the whole thing before they swap round. I think it's likely that that this will stay as a fantasy – pity!

What's your most memorable sexual encounter?
Mmmm, it involved my mate's little brother; yes he was legal and a randy little bastard. It was when we met up with him in a local nightclub. He turned me on so much just looking at him. I was with someone at the time, but in the end I couldn't resist any more. So I went up to him and whispered in his ear, 'If I was single I'd f*** your brains out!' I

walked off calmly and he just stood there stunned. As he didn't react immediately, I started to lose interest. I thought he was too shy for me. But a bit later in the evening, he came up behind me, grabbed my hand and dragged me to a dark corner. My boyfriend was in the club, so we were taking risks, but I think that gave it more of a buzz.

It was hot, steamy and dark in the club and we were rubbing up against each other so fiercely we may as well have been f***ing! It was the best virtual f*** I have ever had. I had to have more of him, so I rang him a few days later and we finished where we left off, about nine times to be precise. It had to end though, as it was getting dangerous. He also had a girlfriend and I couldn't deal with all the deceit.

What do you think about group sex? Have you tried it?

I haven't tried it, although I do enjoy thinking/fantasising about it. But I think I'd get too jealous if I saw my partner getting it on with another woman.

I'm friends with two couples and they all did it together. It's kinda f***ed up their friendship and made it uncomfortable for them to be around each other for a while. So I guess I would be up for it if my partner was not involved, he, he!

TELL ME A SECRET

What advice would you give to someone who wanted to get into this business?

I'd say, don't take yourself too seriously and you must be able to handle rejection – lots of it! Invest in a good cleanser, as your skin will get shitty from all that pore-blocking slap you have to wear! Also, have fun and make as many new friends and contacts as poss. In this business, white lies are cool! Age, bra size, height, experience for the job. They are all allowed! Finally, send your photos out everywhere. You never know whose hands they could fall into!

Which bloke do you fancy the most?

Robbie Williams, Ashton Kutchner, Ryan Phillipe, Jared Leto, Freddie Ljungberg, Stephen Dorff, Johnny Dep ... And , Posh, don't worry, because Becks does nothing for me!!!!

Tell me a secret ... The first time I tried speed I was 15 and it was with my best mate. We were bored of drinking MD 20/20 and experimenting with marijuana, so this seemed like it could be fun. We paid a fiver for a gram off some kid who lived down the street from me.

I must point out that I am being completely honest in reiterating these events, although it may come across that I am talking about drugs in a

NIKITA

positive way. This is not the case – I just want to explain how I felt at the time and in no way am I condoning illegal drugs at all.

As I was saying, we took half a gram each and waited. Then we 'came up'. It was quite a nice feeling. Not like when you take pills or LSD. With speed you are completely aware of everything that is going on. Every song sounds fantastic, and you are a great dancer, a confident speaker. We stayed up all night chatting. I thought how could this drug be harmful?

The next day was a different story. I didn't actually get to sleep till 8am. Well, I didn't really sleep at all. I just forced my eyes shut and tossed and turned. By mid-afternoon I was really ill. I couldn't move. My whole body ached and was stiff. I was really emotional and tearful and when I tried to go to the loo it was as though my guts had fallen out of my body. I later learned that this horrid stomach upset was common and was referred to as 'gut rot'. Eating was the last thing on my mind. Just looking at food made me feel sick. My mouth was sore and ulcerated and I couldn't even drink water. I took comfort in sipping a carton of Five Alive. It took me six hours to sip the whole carton! Welcome to my first 'come down'. But being a naïve 15-year-old, I just put this horrid experience down to it being my first time. The following weekend we did it again, but this time we bought a gram each.

My mum and dad are very good parents and were very strict disciplinarians with me, but it's hard to keep a tight reign on a 15-year-old. I had a curfew of midnight, which was way earlier than most of my friends. But, like most typical 15-year-olds, I was moody and hated being around my family.

When I wasn't hanging out on the local estate with my friends I was in my room playing Super Mario Brothers till the early hours. So it was normal for me to sleep till midday at the weekends. Also, I did a lot of drug experimentation on nights I knew I would be sleeping over at a friend's, so my parents didn't notice any strange behaviour. I had a big attitude problem anyway and I used to talk to my mother like shit. So the nights that she'd catch me climbing out my bedroom window at 3am, because I was still buzzing, she would put down to me just being rebellious. I was always a sensible child when I was younger, so the last thing on my parents' minds was that I was involved with drugs.

Very quickly after I started doing speed, I started taking the drug on school nights. I began truanting and falling asleep behind the school stage to recover from my 'come downs'.

I eventually worked out that there was a good

way to escape the dreaded 'comedown' and that was, basically, you had to take more. Soon I was taking a few dabs before my lessons. No one noticed. I didn't really ever do anything out of character on speed. I just became more confident, enthusiastic and energetic. By this time my friend had dropped out of school and I was truanting so much my teachers were sending letters home.

My weight was only six stone. I hardly ate. But people always knew me as skinny anyway. Again, it was something that no one picked up on. I always made sure I wore baggy clothes, which hid how skinny I was. One particular favourite item of clothing was my grey Fruit Of The Loom sweatshirt that would fit a grown man. I think I've still got it at home somewhere.

Eventually I went from taking one gram to two grams to taking pure base (speed that is supposedly stronger as it hasn't been cut with glucose and all sorts of other household crap). I also took pink champagne – that was speed that had a slight pink tinge to it. I liked speed as it lasted way longer than cocaine. It was cheap as hell and you could take it anywhere and everywhere. On a downside, it tasted like shit. Possibly the worst taste ever – so I overcome that by bombing it (wrapping it in a rizla and swallowing the rizla so it explodes in your belly like a little 'bomb'). Sometimes I'd snort it. I once snorted a gram straight out of the wrap without cutting it and smoothing out all the lumps. My nose was a right mess the next day. When I think back I can't believe I was so sick and depraved. I'd even put it in my tea. It got to a point where I was buying quantities big enough to deal but they were just for my own consumption.

I once tried to cheat by cutting it with glucose to make double the amount and sell it on. I put red food colouring in it to pass it off as pink champagne to get more cash, but I ended up f***ing the whole lot up. It didn't matter though as I'd eaten it all by the end of the week.

By the time I was 17 I had a bit of a reputation of being a 'whizz head'. I wasn't the only one. The estate that we lived on was a bit rough and practically everyone was on speed at one time. Once my neighbour and I stole her flatmate's TV and video and sold it to Cash Converters so we could go and 'get on it'.

At this time I'd also experimented with pills and GHB, which I can't really remember much about as I was usually on speed when I took them anyway. One night at a hardcore rave in Stevenage I put 8 grams into a bottle of coke and downed it, then topped it off with a couple of pills. That night I was so ill. My mate, Mark, found me in a right state on the floor in the toilets. I refused to see the paramedics in case they pumped my stomach and, even worse, they would tell my parents. So I begged Mark to stay with me outside the rave. We sat together for five hours with me rocking backwards and forwards, making the odd whimper, while he gave me sips of water, trying to keep me alert.

It was the day after that night that I decided to sort out my mess of a life. Yeah, I'd done well at school and had just completed a first year of A levels in Art, English and German. But my life was more important. If I stayed in the area, I knew I'd end up in the gutter. So I dropped my German A level in a suitcase, packed my English coursework, my sketch pad, pencils and Indian ink and went to stay with relatives in Cyprus. My parents agreed this would be good for me, as I was a bit of a wild child and thought that some time away would keep me from getting into trouble.

Being in Cyprus was a breath of fresh air. I couldn't get any drugs at all out there. I felt naturally refreshed. My appetite returned and I started to put on weight. A month later I weighed a healthy eight-and-a-half stone. I came home, completed my A levels and avoided my old friends like the plague. As soon as my exams were over I went straight back out to Cyprus for my 18th birthday – this time with my parents. It was really weird, but being in Cyprus and learning to feel clear headed and confident without taking speed made me realise that speed wasn't addictive for me at all.

It wasn't all great. I did suffer from panic attacks and nausea for a long time afterwards and now, even at the age of 24, I still get panic attacks, which I believe are a result of the amount of mental damage I did to myself.

Nowadays, I won't even drink any more than one Smirnoff ice at a time – let alone take any substance that will alter my perceptions or intoxicate me. I'm very lucky I escaped a possible worse fate.

My parents agreed that when I came back from Cyprus I was altogether a much nicer person, but they couldn't exactly pinpoint why. Only I knew the real reason. Since then I have told my mum that I had experimented with drugs in my teens. But she doesn't know to what extent. I've spared my dad the details, as it would disappoint him so much.

I have never shared this with anyone and, when my parents do read this, I hope that they will not be too ashamed of what I did. I want them to be proud of the fact that I fought the problem head on. It's because of my parents love, support and the way they raised me that made me strong enough to get over this and make a success out of my life. Thanks Mum and Dad.

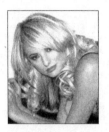

TORI

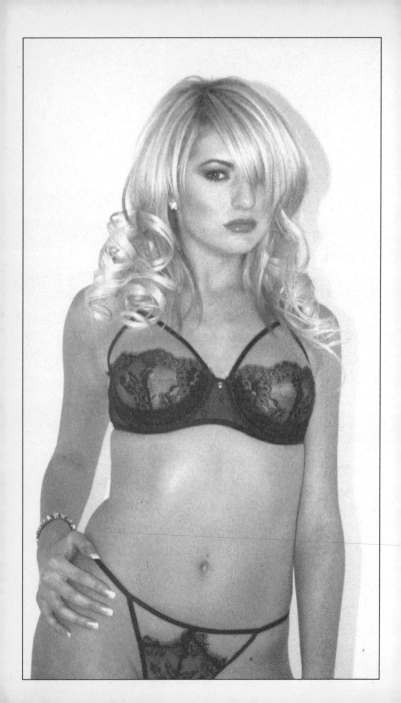

TORI

Name: Victoria Taylor
Model/Dance Name: Tori
Star Sign: Aries
Age: 19
Vital Stats: 34B - 24 - 34
Lives: Hull, East Yorkshire
Fave Food: Mexican
Fave Drink: Champagne, of course!

Where do you work?
I work worldwide – depends on what the project is and how much it is paying!

I have done work for the *Star*, *Daily Sport*, *Max Power* and have appeared in other magazines like *Nuts* etc.

How did you get into modelling?
It was something I always wanted to do. I made

the mistake of telling everyone at school that I wanted to be a model, which gave them an excuse to tease and pick on me. They said that I was too skinny to be a model and took the piss out of me because I was ambitious. 'You will never make it as a model,' they used to shout. They branded me a slag, because they assumed anyone who wanted to take their clothes off for a living must sleep around – 'Well, hello, 18-year-old mother-of-four, look at me now! I'm a working model who's got here herself!'

I hated all the teasing at school, but now, thanks to being teased, it's made me stronger and more determined to be a success – I've got the last laugh, because I'm the one living my dream.

It hasn't been easy by any means. I spent, and still spend, hours/days researching, making as many contacts as I can and entering every competition. It has to be like that at first, until you have reached the level when you have an agent and PR team behind you. You have to fight for every opportunity.

I got my big break when I had just turned 17. It was my first holiday in Ayia Napa, Cyprus. I was there with my boyfriend, Andrew Newton – he played Robbie Flynn in *Hollyoaks*. We were chilling at a beach bar, indulging in our first beer of the day, when the *Sport* newspaper spotted me.

TORI

I lied and said I was 18 and got some work. It all went from there really. I have never stopped working since.

I don't think people realise that it is hard work and only the very determined and ambitious make it. You work long hours and are expected to look glamorous ALL the time. Don't even get me started on the mental strain and frustration – the last five years I've been told I'm a wannabe, a marriage wrecker, been compared to the Kiss 'n' Tell Queen, Alicia Davail – but, God, do I love this career and wouldn't change my life for anything!

What's the biggest fee/tip you have ever earned?
£6,000 for a Kiss 'n' Tell.

What highstreet publications have you been in? Have you worked with any famous people?
I have been in the *Star*, the *Sport*, *News of the World*, *Max Power* and most of the middle-shelf lad mags such as *Nuts* etc.

What other work have you done?
I used to be a travel agent. I only worked there so I could get cheap holidays – every other weekend to Magaluf (shagaluf) – everyone loves Magaluf, cheap beer and easy sex!!

TELL ME A SECRET

Do you have any famous friends?
Everyone is everyone's friend in this business, that's all the fun of it! Callum Best (George Best's son) is a sweet guy but, like I said, it's a close circle and everyone shags everyone!

I've caught up with the band Blue quite a few times lately. I got chatting to them on yet another holiday to Cyprus. We all went to a club and got really drunk. Not long after I got back from Cyprus I bumped into them again at a concert. We all had a really good laugh, they are all good guys and know how to enjoy themselves – that's all I have to say about Blue, nothing more happened, honest!

What does your family think of the work you do?
Nothing suprises my mum. At the age of six I was posing in the garden starkers, practising my glamour poses. At nine I used to tell my dad I was going to be a stripper – so I think they knew it was coming. They are really supportive. I remember when I won a competition in the *Star* and my mum was really proud and spent hours ringing all her friends and family to gloat about her daughter's triumph.

Friends are a total different kettle of fish. You find out very quickly who are your true friends. I have fallen out with a lot of my friends over my career, but I just think 'tough shit'. I see them

TORI

collecting their dole on a Monday morning and just laugh to myself – 'who are they to judge what I do? At least I'm doing something with my career'.

What's your funniest moment?
I had just been at the *Max Power* show at Birmingham NEC. It had been a long stint and I couldn't wait to get into my comfy clothes. I was with my photographer, Nick, who had a hot date that night. We jumped straight into the car in my modelling gear and I decided to get changed in the car. I climbed into the back of the car, totally stripped off, top and all. Almost completely naked, apart from a bit of string! I bent down to grab my clothes and when I popped back up, to my surprise I had an audience – a coach full of footie supporters. They were all squashed up against the window, cheering me on. Now I'm not a shy girl! So, rather than squirm with embarrassment, I just waved my hands in the air, giving them a free full-on view of my boobs. Nick, who was driving the car, didn't find it funny at all. As he realised what was going on, he squirmed with embarrassment, put his foot down and zoomed off down the motorway – spoilsport!

What's your scariest moment?
I had got a job at a car show at the NEC. There

was about four thousand people in attendance, most of them men. My job was to parade about on a stage half-naked, making the cars look more sexy and appealing. I don't think I have ever been so nervous. I felt physically sick. My adrenaline was through the roof, I thought I might have a heart attack. All kind of things were going through my mind – what if I throw up on the stage or get stagefright and just stand there like a twat? I got my call and headed to the stage, still shaking. As soon as I faced my audience the nerves completely disappeared and I got the biggest buzz in my life ... yeah, even a bigger buzz than mind-blowing sex!

Have you ever turned down work and why?
Oh, God, yes – I'm always turning work down. There are some sick perverts out there – had lots of dodgy offers for full-on legs-open nudity (*Hustler* magazine) ... NO THANK YOU!

Do you have a sexual fantasy?
I would love to be laid in a Jacuzzi with five or six brunettes totally naked. The thought of it actually really turns me on. We would have lots of fun in the water, fondling each other and rubbing our soapy breasts together would be sheer heaven. Then I would like to pick one of the brunettes,

who would most definitely be Jerri Bryne – she is pure lush.

What's your most memorable sexual encounter?
No, I can't tell you, it's far too rude. I would love to tell you and you would absolutely love it, but it's just too rude. I'm blushing just thinking about it.

What do you think about group sex? Have you tried it?
Yes, I think it's fine – as long as everyone's happy, then it's OK. I don't think it would work if you're pressurised into it, or if you share a secure relationship. I s'pose a bit of porn could start the excitement off for threesomes. Personally, I've never done swapping round partners – I'd get too jealous. I like my man all to myself – I'm a very loyal kinda girl.

What advice would you give to someone who wanted to get into this business?
A model needs to have lots of things; firstly she needs to have belief in herself and the confidence to succeed. She needs independence and ambition, which also plays an important part in the success of your career and a major factor as to whether you will in fact make it in the business.

TELL ME A SECRET

I always make sure I look after myself well. It doesn't have to be that you work out at the gym each day, just simple things like, drink lots of water and always moisturise.

Which bloke do you fancy the most?
I wouldn't mind a slice of Prince William or Harry – or both!

Tell me a secret ... My life was going great, I had a boyfriend, Andrew Newton, from *Hollyoaks*, who I loved and, if I'm honest, still love very much. My career was just starting to kick off and, generally, everything seemed to be going in the right direction.

I thought Andrew was my soulmate, and I didn't want to think of life without him. I thought he felt the same. He promised me a lot of things, but six months down the line he was part of the London party scene. I was only managing part-time modelling so I was still working for a travel agent on the Bransholme Council Estate in Hull.

I use to dread looking through the newspapers and magazines. Each week he would be splashed all over the papers with the likes of Brooke Kinsella from *Eastenders*, Jodie Marsh and Abbi Titmus, to name a few.

I used to get pissed off with being made a fool

of and, well, you know, a woman scorned and all that! I decided to cash in on it. As people said at the time, I sold my soul, but, believe me, £6,000 for a Kiss 'n' Tell is good money. I did the Kiss 'n' Tell, which led to another Kiss 'n' Tell and another. I didn't care any more and neither did he.

I think everyone knows these kinds of stories might start as a bit of revenge, but mostly they are to boost careers. But sometimes you have to live with the media exploiting the information you give to them.

After all this, I did learn not to trust reporters, after one made me sound like an over possessive freak and really pathetic. I can honestly say I learned from Andrew's mistakes. In this industry you have to be so careful, as people are quick to judge and they enjoy seeing people's careers go down the pan – after all, it makes good reading. I truly believe Andrew was a blessing in my life. If it weren't for him, I wouldn't have as much determination to go on after all this crap. It's a shame it ended as it did. I do miss him. I miss the good times we had together. I still think he is my soulmate, but I guess sometimes things aren't meant to be.

During the time I was angry with Andrew and still wanting to get revenge for the torment he put me through, I was invited to what promised to be a great party at the Brit Awards. I remember I was feeling particularly good that day. I had lots of modelling jobs on offer and, at last, things seemed to be turning around for me. I was getting a good reputation and was partying every night and enjoying life as a whole. However, this party ended up being a very interesting night indeed – and until now I have not shared exactly what happened.

I took my friend, Sarah, along to the party. Bless her, she had never been out of Hull before, so this night was a big shock to her. I had booked us in to a hotel in Kensington. Soon after checking in we were downing the contents of the mini-bar.

We were having such a great time at the Brit Awards and we were in high spirits when we reached the after-party, which was at the Kensington Roof Top Gardens.

We were dancing away and getting very drunk on champagne. I moved over to the bar for another glass of champagne. I saw this guy who was blond, tanned and whom I noticed had been eyeing me up all night. He finally made his move on me at the bar and asked if I would like a drink. He seemed to be out with a group of guys, but I wasn't taking much notice. Of course, I didn't turn down the drink and ordered a glass of champagne. I was hoping that he would buy a

TORI

bottle to share, but no, he literally just got me a glass – a bit tight I thought for someone who looked like he had a few bob!

We chatted for ages. We had obviously clicked and soon we moved on to the dance floor. It was then he kissed me. We were dancing very close; he was touching my body and before I knew it he grabbed me hard and gave me a full-on snog, pressing his body up against mine. I let him snog me, after all he was pretty cute – not my usual type, but scored high on the cute factor.

About 30 minutes after our initial snog, I went to the ladies to reapply my lippy as he had kissed most of it off! No sooner had I hit the loos than a reporter, who said she worked for the *News of the World*, approached me and said, 'Do you know that's James Beattie?'

I looked blank at her, thinking, James who? 'He plays for England', she continued, 'and he has a girlfriend.'

I didn't really care, I was having fun and was very pissed by this stage. I just shrugged, slapped my lippy on and headed back for another glass of champagne.

When I got back to the table, James was waiting for me with a bottle of champagne. We drank it like it was water. I remember at one point we were drinking from the bottle.

TELL ME A SECRET

Not long after we had finished off the bottle of champagne, we decided to make a dash and disappear from the party. I remember someone was shouting at him, I think it was either an agent or some PR person. Whoever they were, they were obviously pissed at him. They were telling him not to leave, but he didn't care.

We had to leave through the back doors so as not to be seen. He held on to my hand as we made our way very drunkenly down lots of stairs – I had to stop I was knackered. He then picked me up and was kissing me. His hands were all over my body and, to be honest, I remember it was a struggle to keep his hands off me. It was then I started to think he wasn't really all that nice and was a bit pushy, but I wanted to leave the party. My friend had already left and I didn't want to go back into the party on my own.

We grabbed a cab outside with a few of his mates. As the cab set off, he put his head out of the window and started shouting out at passers-by – I remember thinking what a dickhead.

We got out at the Funky Buddha. He jumped to the front of the queue and they refused his entry, so we had to wait for about 15 minutes before we got in and they made him pay. He kicked off again about having to pay – it was only a tenner, and it was really embarrassing.

TORI

Once I was in the club, I bumped into Callum Best and ended up snogging Callum – he was much, much better than James. After going from one to the other, I told James I wanted to leave. I think he thought 'go back together', but there was no way I was going to go back to my hotel with him. I've never been easy and wasn't going to start, especially with someone I wasn't that keen on. Besides I wasn't going to be another notch on a footballer's bedpost, particularly after sampling his kisses I didn't think I would be missing a great deal!

I've not seen him since, but I did hear that him and his girlfriend split up, guess she found out what he was really like – lucky escape I say!

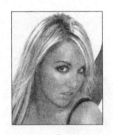

DANNII

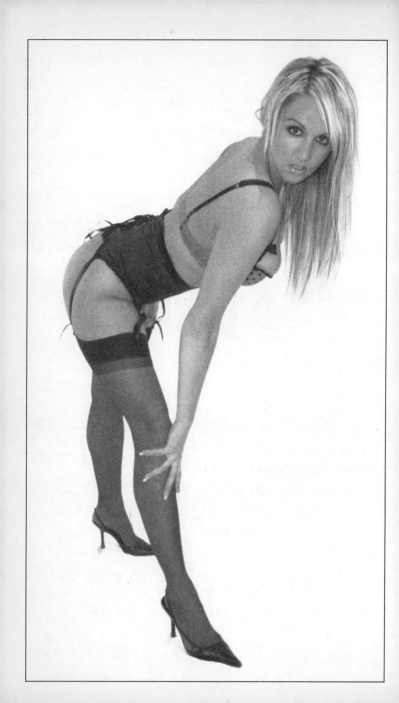

DANNII

Name: Dannii Harwood
Model/Dance Name: Dannii
Star Sign: Gemini
Age: 22
Vital Stats: 34D-26-36
Lives: Epsom
Fave Food: Mushy peas
Fave Drink: Stella Artois

Where do you work?
I am a professional glamour model and have been modelling since early 2004. While my preferred work is glamour photo shoots and live appearances at events, such as *Max Power*, it is necessary to take on other work such as promotional and hospitality work, as well as drama and dance tuition, in order to pay the bills. To date my work has taken me to Italy, Spain and

the Netherlands, but the majority is UK based, predominantly in the South East.

How did you get into modelling?

I was trained at Laine Theatre Arts School and I am a professional dancer and qualified teacher. I also studied musical theatre. This formed the major part of my career prior to taking up modelling on a full-time basis earlier in 2004.

It started when a friend recommended me for my first modelling assignment. She had many years' experience and had appeared on Page 3 etc. She had started an agency of her own and I was one of her first models. I had previously done some fashion modelling on an occasional basis, but never really knew if I had what it takes to go full-time. She convinced me that I could make it in the glamour industry, even though, at the time, topless was not an option.

My first big break was as the new face of Golden Tee Golf, including a poster campaign and a live appearance at the British Masters, where I met with the Ryder Cup golfers. One of the golfers even asked me out on a date.

My face started to appear in pubs all over the country, and it was a great feeling to be recognised as I walked into a bar.

DANNII

I have to say that first assignment felt wicked and that's what got me hooked.

What's the biggest fee/tip you have ever earned?
During a hospitality job at the Dorchester Hotel, I was offered (genuinely) £10,000 to spend one night with a top, well-known businessmen. There were many other famous names at this function, most of who were also offering similar money. One of the guys manages a football club; the other is a big noise in the city of London. Just in case you were wondering – yes, I turned the offer down!

What highstreet publications have you been in? Have you worked with any famous people?
My first media print job was for the *Sunday People* and I was interviewed by the infamous Garry Bushell. This was following the *Test the Nation* TV programme in which I appeared as one of the 40 models taking part. The shoot was at Canary Wharf with Martin Spaden. The booking was through one of my agents who has still not paid me. A lesson learned!

I have since appeared in various magazines including *FHM*, *Revs*, *Max Power* and most recently *Ice*. The *Ice* shoot was with Jens of Popstars Ltd and took place in King's Cross. I am also set to appear in *Front* and *Maxim* in the coming months.

What other work have you done?
As a professional dancer I have done various jobs, ranging from a backing dancer for a Kylie Minogue tribute band to choreographing a show at the London Palladium.

Do you have any famous friends?
I used to go to school with Catherine Zeta Jones, although she is a few years older. Her mum used to make my dance costumes. I also worked with and am still friends with, Lee Latchford Evans, from Steps. I was in pantomime with him for two years.

I have made many friends since being on the model circuit and have been seen with Prince Harry, Frank Lampard and was asked out by Scott Sullivan (Jordan's and Jodie's ex) – I turned him down!

What does your family think of the work you do?
Although they would not stop me from pursuing my chosen career, they have made it clear that they would have preferred me to continue my dancing work.

One issue that is a difficult discussion point is whether I will do topless work. At present I have not, but as the offers roll in it is something that I am considering. However, I am very aware of my family's feelings and this is making my decision even more difficult.

I have always wanted to do something that would make my mum proud and not be ashamed to show her friends. Lots of thinking to do on this one!

What's your funniest moment?

One of my funniest moments started through an enquiry, which I received via my website www.dannii-harwood.com. It was for a nude photo shoot. Several emails later, having explained that I would only work up to implied nude, we came to the question of whether I was 'fully trimmed'. I replied that it did not matter, as I did not do nude. He insisted on knowing, as it affected the underwear shots he was planning. In the end I admitted to being 'trimmed'.

I took down the address, which I thought was great because it was close by. It was only when I got there I realised it was my local gym, which I visit about four times a week, I was really embarrassed as I was greeted by some of the guys I regularly work out with. They have never let me forget it.

The things we go through to get work!

TELL ME A SECRET

What's your scariest moment?

My worst experience was attending a shoot with someone who made out he was a photographer. He knew that I only would do implied topless. He seemed to think that this agreement of implied nude was not important once I arrived at the shoot. As time went on, it became clear that he was expecting me to go much further, culminating in me performing oral sex on him while he filmed me. I made it perfectly clear where he could shove his camera! Fortunately, my chaperone was in the next room and came to my rescue before anything happened. You really have to check these guys out first, and I am much more careful now.

Have you ever turned down work and why?

I have turned down numerous jobs that required nude and beyond, including Page 3 at the start of my career. The biggest of these was the £10,000 'job' offer at the Dorchester that I previously mentioned.

Do you have a sexual fantasy?

Being pulled out of the audience by Liam Gallagher and letting him seduce me on stage in front of the audience. I would love to live this out but I think his wife would get a bit jealous. Or maybe her sexual fantasy might be to watch!

DANNII

What's your most memorable sexual encounter?
Joining the Mile-high Club, I must have orgasmed five times (it must be the altitude). On leaving the toilet, I received a standing ovation from the passengers. I think there were a few questions from the children to their parents.

What do you think about group sex? Have you tried it?
I have tried it once and would not mind another, maybe a threesome with Britney Spears and Liam Gallagher. It was fun the first time and I would recommend it!

What advice would you give to someone who wanted to get into this business?
Don't walk away from your previous career immediately and, preferably, keep a part-time job. The work is not always regular and there will be some tough times ahead.

The support of your family is essential and their feelings should always be taken into account when considering the work you undertake.

You should always be prepared to turn work down, however short of money you are. Standards must be maintained and you will regret doing dodgy jobs at a later date.

TELL ME A SECRET

Which bloke do you fancy the most?
Liam Gallagher/Ian Brown/Jude Law.

Tell me a secret ... I have had a great secret for years. The memories of my secret sexy naughtiest night ever are as fresh in my mind as the day it happened. I am sure that anyone that has shared a similar experience would say the same.

It was one of those hot sticky summer nights that we don't get very often, but when we do, something always seems to happen. The night we were out partying at Trap Nightclub in Wardour Street, Epsom, proved to be no exception. I had gone to the club, with my now ex-boyfriend and a group of his mates. I had not been with my boyfriend for very long, although, as a group, we had all known each other for a few years and were good mates. I was not sure how committed I was to the relationship, and my feeling was that it was unlikely to be a long-lasting one, but you never know.

As the night went on we got hotter and hotter. The air conditioning in the club was struggling to keep us cool. As a result, we drank more and more as the evening went on. Eventually it got so hot that we decided to carry on the party back at – let's call them – Neil and Steve's house. They were two brothers from our group, who shared a house together. I had fancied Steve some time ago and he had asked me out, but I had just finished a long-term relationship and was not ready for another so I declined his offer. That didn't stop me still fancying him though.

By the time we got near Steve and Neil's house, the drink had taken its toll on some of our mates and they had drifted off home. My boyfriend also wanted to head off home, as he had work the next day. I wanted to carry on partying and felt ready for anything; as far as I was concerned, the night was still young.

I argued with my boyfriend for a while, but in the end he went home to bed and I went back to Steve and Neil's house. By the time we got there, it was just the three of us left. Although I had known them for some time, I suddenly felt a little awkward as I was the only girl.

Not long after we got back to the house Steve opened the bubbly, the music went on and we started dancing and having a good laugh. We then started to play drinking games like truth or dare, and the conversation inevitably got on to the subject of sex. I was getting really horny talking about sex with two attractive guys.

The mood of the music changed and some slow tracks came on. I took it in turns to dance with Steve and Neil. As time went on I was really getting in the mood, particularly with Steve, as I had fancied him for a while, although both brothers were extremely fit and good looking.

It was now the early hours of the morning and the drink had started to make Neil feel sleepy. Steve and I were still wide awake. Neil went to make coffee and Steve and I carried on dancing and getting closer. I could feel his hands all over me. I wanted him.

Although I was loving every minute of it, my emotions were all over the place. I was going out with someone who I liked, but realistically was not going to be with long term and here I was with someone that I had really fancied for some time, but I had convinced myself that I did not want a long-term relationship.

I had drunk far too much and my thoughts were irrational. I generally think of myself as someone who is faithful. Even when I had been tempted in the past, I had never succumbed to unfaithfulness but, on this occasion, I decided to go for it. Just as we were about to kiss, Neil walked back in with the coffee.

It was as though someone had switched a light off. All the electricity that had built up between us went flat. The three of us sat around talking about the early part of the evening and laughing at the events and friends

DANNII

that had got up and made idiots of themselves on the dance floor.

Then the temperature seemed to be going up rather than cooling down. It must have been the humidity, as I was getting really hot and feeling sticky. Steve and I went outside to get some air. This is where he first kissed me. We were snogging for a while on the deck outside the back door. The air was hot and did nothing to cool me off. I just wanted to get out of my clothes.

Neil called out and told us that he was going to bed and wished us a VERY good night. This was just what I had in mind! I had fantasised for the last couple of hours about what was going to happen and where, but things don't always turn out as you plan.

Steve took me by the hand and we went back into the lounge. He put the slow music back on. We resumed our dance positions and his hands returned to where he had them before Neil disturbed us with the coffee. Steve was now unzipping my dress and easing it off my shoulders. I did nothing to stop him. My dress then fell to the floor and I kicked it away. Steve's attention then turned to my bra. He seemed to be an expert and I hardly noticed it being undone. I had yet to respond but felt that it was time to show my intentions, so I slowly unbuttoned his shirt. At this point we stumbled towards the sofa and Steve started to remove his trousers.

I was sitting there with just my thong on, when I heard the lounge door creak. I turned my head to see Neil poking his head around the door. He looked a little taken aback and then went bright red. He could not take his eyes off my near-naked body. He stuttered, 'Oh, God, sorry, guys.' However, instead off walking away, he gathered his thoughts and said to Steve, 'You lucky bastard.' I laughed and asked Neil if he liked what he saw. He simply replied 'stunning'.

A little smirk came across my face and Steve asked me what was so funny. I turned to Steve and whispered in his ear 'Would you mind if Neil joined in?'

To my surprise and delight, he said, 'Not at all, us brothers should stick together.'

I walked across the room to a bemused Neil. I don't think he knew where to look. I took him by the hand and led him back to the sofa. I sat him at the opposite end to Steve and I sat down between them. By now Neil was starting to catch on and he started to take his shirt off. Sandwiched between them I put one arm around each of them. I could not believe that this was really happening. I was feeling very naughty and adventurous, not like anything that I had experienced before.

As I had one arm around each of them, they naturally moved closer. I was giggling deep inside as they took hold of a breast each. For the rest of that night I made love to two beautiful men and loved every moment of it. The whole experience can only be described as surreal.

This had been my secret fantasy and I was fortunate enough to fulfil it.

Although the whole experience was wild and fantastic, it did not lead to a relationship with either of the guys. The inevitable happened with my boyfriend – we split up but it was nothing to do with my night of fun.

I often see the brothers when we meet up with our group of friends and we exchange the odd smile and a wink. We have never discussed it with each other, or told anyone about it. We agreed that it would remain a secret between the three of us – Ooops!

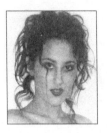

KAT

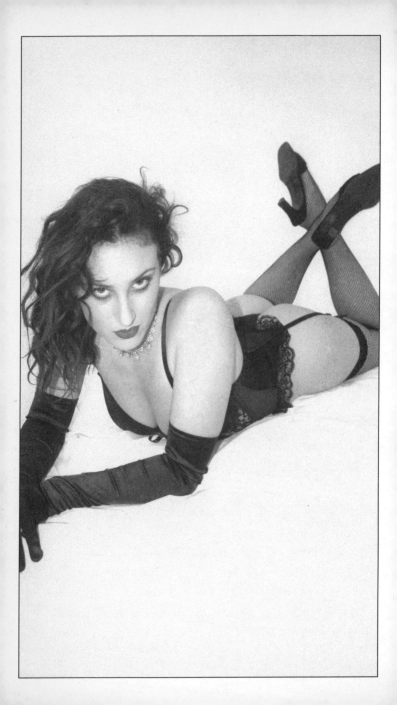

KAT

Model/Dance Name: Kat Ballie
Star Sign: Pisces
Age: 20
Vital Stats: 34DD-24-34
Lives: In a van I so move around - originally from Portsmouth
Fave Food: Chocolate muffins
Fave Drink: Hot chocolate

Where do you work?

My work takes me all over the UK. I live in a mobile home, so I live wherever work takes me. I didn't originally set out to live in a mobile home; it's just how things turned out.

I used to be based in Allaway Avenue, Paulsgrove, until the landlord sold the flat from underneath us. I really liked living in my two-bedroom flat. We had been there for just under a year and felt very settled. But the flat was sold and we had only a short time to find another home. Our only income was from doing a bit of magic and modelling. We didn't have any regular cash coming in and decent accommodation was very hard to come by.

Paul, my partner, and I had allotments at Portchester and enjoyed being close to our friends and family. One day when we were on our way home from Brighton, frantically thinking about where we would find another home, we found a little basset hound. It was a lovely little thing and distracted us from all the crap of finding a flat.

We knew she must belong to someone, so we searched high and low for her owner and left our phone number in local shops in the area. When we had no luck, we decided we would keep her. We set off to find a pet shop to get a lead, which proved to be more difficult than we thought – what pet shops open on a Sunday at 4pm?

We started our journey back to Portsmouth with our new little friend. During the journey we had a long discussion about how we were going to find a new rented flat with a dog. It was difficult enough but we now had the added pressure of another mouth to feed and a landlord's nightmare. I don't know whether we

KAT

were just ill-fated or just complete f***-wit's! Our work in magic and modelling took us all over the country, so we decided that the simple answer would be to get a caravan.

Later that day the dog's owner phoned and was reunited with her little bassett. We also found out that she worked in the music industry so we gave her my demo. Fate, eh?

Even without the dog we still thought that a mobile home would be a good decision. We found a great caravan, a 16-foot Colchester, and are keeping our eyes peeled for a dog that needs a good home to add to our existing little family, me, Paul and Marley our cat.

The first place we stayed at with our caravan was Cinder Hill farm in Horsted Keynes. It was very pretty and our neighbours were a field of sheep. The best thing about being in the caravan is the feeling of being free and waking up in a field surrounded by nature. It's also got to be the best place I've stayed at as it was the place we did all of our learning and adjusting. I was TV- and internet-deprived for a week. With all that extra time I learned that there was more to do and enjoy than sitting on my bum watching telly. I went out picking fruit and on bike rides, went on the Bluebell line and went skating. I even had my friend, Aimie, come to stay.

It is great fun being carefree and we always manage to find different work wherever we go. The best thing about being in a caravan is, if we don't like the area, or don't like the work, we move on.

How did you get into modelling?

I always wanted to be a model or a singer from a very early age. I loved being on stage. I started dancing at the age of five and learned tap, ballet, modern and jazz at the 'Stardust Dance Troupe' in Copnor Portsmouth. I did my first dance show at the age of six. A few of the places I performed were the Theatre Royal in Portsmouth and the Kings Theatre in Southsea.

I did my first catwalk show in Cascades shopping centre Portsmouth with 'Stardust', aged 12 and no one recognised me from school. I looked great. That year I also joined my first band 'Afterglo'. We got a couple of reviews in *Venue* magazine and performed in many pubs like the Contented Pig, The Air Balloon and the Kingston Tavern in North End.

After I returned from being on the run (I will explain later), I found myself with money from the press and TV interviews. This paid for a portfolio to be done with a studio called TVP in Swindon, with a guy called Bob, who I found in the Yellow

KAT

Pages. I was 16 at the time, so I lied about my age to get it done. After my portfolio was done we carried on shooting together with a TFP (Time For Prints – no money is exchanged, but the model gets photos for her portfolio and the photographer gets pics for his) arrangement. He said I was a natural and I learned a lot over those months. I decided on my modelling levels, which would, and still do, go up to tasteful nudes.

My first job was with Matt Evans from Creamtop, when I was 16. I found him advertising for models in *The Stage*. I called him and arranged a shoot. I was quite nervous, but I knew I was perfectly safe as Paul was with me. We did a couple of hours' glamour and I'm not quite sure what I was paid, but it was over £100. I left the shoot feeling fantastic and on a high. I couldn't wait to see the photos, which he had promised to email me.

After every shoot I found myself collecting better images and I would upload them on to sites and advertise myself and still do. Most of my work comes from sites I'm on such as 'Be Seen Here' and 'Model Heaven'. Photographers will see my pages and then email me or call. I also get a lot of work through going to events and doing magic shows. If I do a magic show I'm sure to get modelling work and vice versa.

TELL ME A SECRET

What's the biggest fee/tip ypu have ever earned?
My biggest modelling fee was £200. It was for three hours topless modelling for a poster campaign for Steve from Mbt in the Isle of Wight.

What other highstreet publications have you been in?
I have been in both the *Mirror* and the *Mail*. I also do a lot of magazine work, such as *Loaded* October 2004 and *Nuts* November 2004.

What other work have you done?
Currently I'm a full-time entertainer/model. I have done other work along the way. I've been a dry cleaner, and a waitress in The Smoking Dog in Malmesbury. I've also done a lot of telesales work in Portsmouth. I was a sales administrator for a cleaning company in Portsmouth. I used to clean The Mary Rose Museum in Portsmouth and varnished a few floors as well.

But Paul and I decided life was too short and we both packed in our jobs and decided to do what we love to do: magic, singing and modelling. I would never do anything I don't love or enjoy. You see, I'm not into my lifestyle for money, it's a passion. I also value my time more than money and would much rather be broke sometimes than stuck in a job I hated just to get by. We keep our living costs low.

KAT

Apart from the modelling I enjoy going out and doing magic. Essentially, our act is based around fast visual close-up illusions developed on the streets and pubs of Britain when Paul and I were on the run. At first the magic was our lifeline and an anonymous way of making money to stay alive. More recently we have performed at conventions and clubs such as Club Wicked in London and the Fantasy Fayre. It's a very saucy act where I produce cards from revealing places! I'm working on a stage act at the moment, which involves singing, dancing and stripping with a magical cane routine.

I have done magic for Clive from Doctor and the Medics at the Plus Show in Brighton. I couldn't believe how tall he was! He couldn't believe how good we were!

My favourite job has got to be when I did some photos and filming with Charlie and Alice from Paraphotos. They took me to Rivendell Naturist Club in the New Forest; it was fantastic, so relaxed and such a hot day. I spent the afternoon there being photographed and filmed for a DVD called *Alice's Naked Summer*. Charlie and Alice made a wonderful lunch. I spent the afternoon swimming and walking around a beautiful place and got paid for having a great time. It was amazing! They work closely with H&E so keep your eyes out for me.

TELL ME A SECRET

I went to Derrie's house in the middle of the countryside. Derrie was a famous 60s fashion model. She cooked us all a fantastic lunch and I really loved looking at her portfolio. She helped with the clothes, make-up and making the props for the shoot. The end result looked fantastic.

I've worked with Steve from Mbt in Cowes on the Isle of Wight. We worked on creating some great posters. I really liked getting my fluorescence on and standing topless outside a builder's yard. The pictures looked great.

I did a lot of naked work in the woods, which I had the thrill of doing in Crawley, with the guys from the Crawley Camera Club. It's always very funny doing outdoor naked shots, but Paul is always close by with a towel if anyone comes walking past! You usually see their dogs first. Through Andy at the Crawley Camera Club, I did a charity bikini car wash in Brighton, which is where I met Lucie Hide (Miss Brighton) who arranged the event. Miss Essex and loads of other great girls were also there. We had lots of fun washing the cars, getting photos taken and getting the guy from Juice FM Radio station wet.

I also really enjoyed shooting on location with Jim Hellier for a few calendar companies such as Brunel and last year I did some erotic pictures for Alan from The Lady Shop for his stand at Erotica in London. I have lots of great stuff lined up. The work keeps getting better.

When I returned from being on the run I was interviewed by Twiggy and John Leslie for *This Morning*. They were lovely to me. It was amazing to see how the show works. The hair and make-up team were great and they said that, when Paul came out of prison (all will be revealed later), we should come back and show them how happy we are together and I would be able to sing them a song. To date, I still have not received our invite. During the show I had a caller ring in and offer me studio time in Portsmouth, which was wonderful.

Our story was published in every national newspaper and I was the first missing person to be put on the back of a lorry, which I found quite amusing. When I found out we were on *Crime Watch* I was upset because no one had taped it for me! I was asked to do a lot of interviews, most of which I turned down like *Trisha* and *Tonight with Trevor McDonald*. I suppose I just wanted to get on with my life after setting all of the rumours straight with the two exclusives that I did for the *Mirror* and the *Mail*.

When I'm not modelling or doing magic, I'm busy writing and recording songs. When I'm not doing that, I do a lot of promotional work at events like Max Power, Fast and Furious and more recently the Surf Show Expo in Exeter. I also undertake work such as topless waitressing and sales. I suppose you could say I'm an all-round entertainer.

Do you have any famous friends?

I have a few famous porn-star friends. I met Bev Cocks when I was shooting at Starflash studios in Portsmouth. I had heard a lot about her from the studio owner Tom. I had arrived for my shoot and she was just finishing hers. A lot of famous glamour girls have walked through those doors I've been told, such as Jordan and Taylor Paige etc. Bev and I spoke briefly that day and over the months we saw more and more of each other at the studio and we became friends. We bump into each other at events and have a good natter, but as I'm sure you can understand everyone I meet in the industry is busy, busy, busy, so I rarely meet people outside of work.

I did meet Autumn Gothic and Violet Storm when I went to Blueprint in Brighton to do some photos for the *Sport* to advertise The Plus Show. I caught up with them all again at The Plus Show. We sat around in the VIP area, drinking mostly! It must have looked really funny when all of us girls were hanging over the edge of Brighton seafront flashing our boobs and bums! It was a great few days. I also did the Plus stands for 'people like us'. They held the awards for the best porn stars, videos etc ... I still talk a lot to Autumn via email and if I get offers for open-leg or higher levels I pass the photographers on to her.

I have also met Denise Davies, Lorna Morgan and a gangster from *Lock Stock and Two Smoking Barrels* at the show.

At the last Erotica I met Vanessa Feltz, Lelani and a girl from Steps. I was also told Max Clifford was there and Elton John's boyfriend.

What does your family think of the work you do?

I have three families: adopted family, real family and Paul's family. My real family is fantastic and is just as excited as me when a good job comes my way. Paul's family (except for Paul) wishes I was doing something more respectable and generally tell their friends I'm in sales! My adopted family doesn't really bring it up, and Paul, well, he is just glad I'm not doing anything worse.

What's your funniest moment?

My funniest moment while on a job has got to be when I arranged to meet a photographer called Steve in Horsted Keynes, near where my caravan was parked. We drove back to the farm and I showed him all the clothes I had got together for the shoot. He only needed one skirt, top and lots of knickers. After spending years developing poses and facial expressions and spending a long time on my make-up, Paul and I found it hilarious that he only wanted close-up shots of what he called 'my panties'. All the way through the shoot, the usually quiet farm had turned very busy. I was trying to work out how many different and imaginative ways I could flash my gusset! The photographer was very pleased with his photos and wanted to work with me again.

What's your scariest moment?

I guess my scariest moment was when I did a shoot for a photographer. When I arrived at the studio there were two photographers. I was a bit miffed that there were two of them, as I wasn't told beforehand and I would not usually pose naked with two cameras going off at once, due to angles! I work a lot with camera clubs, which is completely different, as they all take their turn and they are all very friendly and welcoming. I didn't sense a relaxed atmosphere at this shoot at all. They both kept trying to touch me and most of all they tried to push me into doing things I didn't want to do, like open-leg shots. Some photographers will try this and when told 'no' they drop it, which didn't happen here at all. I kept professional and did my silent facial conversations with Paul. I do this a lot to let him know that either I'm fine, I'm tired or I'm not happy. If I'm not happy with something Paul will stay close by, and if I'm having fun and I feel safe, then Paul will go and make a cup of tea and chill out. As you can guess he stayed close by. Then they opened up a big case of guns. At first I was a bit worried, as I don't like guns and there was no way I can tell if a gun is real or fake. It just added to the uneasy atmosphere. When I first held the gun I suppose it was a natural reaction to point it at the floor and pull the trigger. I just couldn't help but wonder how and why they had so many guns. I left a few hours later and they were very happy with me. They wouldn't have known I was uneasy as I am always professional and keep a level head.

A few days after the shoot I had an email from a photographer asking me if I had worked for the bloke at the studio. I replied, 'Yes, why? Are you going to be posing for him then?' I joked. He replied, after telling me I was funny, on a more serious note that there was a model who had confided in him, telling him this man had sexually assaulted her. In retrospect, it wasn't such a surprise really.

Another scary moment was when I was driving

back to Chichester from Exeter, where I had been working at the Surf Show. My temperature gauge soared to hot so I pulled off of the road I was on and followed signs to a service station, but when I got there it had been knocked down. I knew I had to stop the car fast and there was nowhere to pull over. I drove to a visible spot in the road and stopped. My 20-year-old Nissan Micra was burning, I could smell it. It was about half an hour away from being dark, my phone battery was running out and about £2 in credit. My car was slap-bang in the middle of a busy road. That was scary! After trying to explain where I was (in the middle of nowhere between Exeter and Chichester) a car came from Cuss Car Care – hooray! A very special thanks to those guys!

Have you ever turned down work and why?

I've turned down all open-leg-work, as I don't think it would do me the best of favours if my singing career comes off. I also think that a sexy, attractive image leaves something to the imagination.

The most ridiculous offer I've had was a bloke offering me £40,000 to be in a film. If it sounds too good to be true it probably is. We spoke and when he couldn't give me names and numbers I politely said goodbye.

KAT

Do you have a sexual fantasy?
To be honest, I don't really have one at the moment and, when I do, it very quickly becomes a reality.

What's your most memorable sexual encounter?
Every time is memorable and it keeps getting better!

What do you think about group sex? Have you tried it?
I am happy with my bloke so it would not interest me, but I don't think there is anything wrong with it if everyone is safe and agrees to it.

What advice would you give to someone who wanted to get into this business?
Try and get together a few snapshots and upload them to a few sites. Then ask if there are any good photographers willing to do TFPs with you. Check their references and always take someone with you. Try and meet as many people as you can in the industry, as networking definitely pays off.

Which bloke do you fancy the most?
Mine!

Tell me a secret ... I think a lot of my current circle of friends will be shocked when they realise who I am. I try and keep my past in the past. I have never even thought of telling the photographers I work with and no one has ever recognised me from the papers. I guess another reason I never talk about it now is that we have moved on and made a life for ourselves and no one would have enough time to hear all the juicy bits. I may write it as a book one day – it would make a great book full of violence, sex, drugs and life on the streets!

It all began when I was 14 and I met this guy, Paul, in a pub. Yeah, I know I was underage but, as I mentioned before, I love singing. Pubs were the only places I could get gigs without too many questions about my age. I was gigging at The Kingston Tavern in Portsmouth. Anyway I got chatting to Paul and we really clicked, love at first sight you could say. He thought I was in my early 20s and I thought he was in his late 20s. I came down to earth with a bit of a bump when one of the band members said that he was a teacher at my school!

When I went back to school the next day I realised that Paul was teaching next door to my tutor room. Paul and I became good friends and I guess we broke the entire teacher-student relationship regs. He would come and watch my gigs and we spoke a lot after school. I found it really easy to share my troubles with him.

I was fed up living at home and being bullied at

school. One day I decided enough was enough and I decided to run away from home. I left for a few days sleeping rough in Southsea. Paul was worried and looked for me high and low. He eventually found me and persuaded me to go home. He took me back to my adoptive parents who rang the police telling them that it was Paul who was to blame, which was the final straw for me. I told Paul I was going and this time for good. He begged me to stay and, when I said no, he told me that if I were going he would have to come too.

I was only 15 and he was my teacher and I knew it was wrong, but we loved each other, so we left. We had a great plan and I'm not sure how but it worked. We had no money and we couldn't use bankcards, as bankcards equalled identities. I had legged it out of the house at the last minute after an argument with my mum in which my room got smashed up and I couldn't find my shoes. I was barefoot and in hardly any clothes. I left with nothing and, as far as I was concerned, I was no one.

At the first opportunity I cut and bleached my hair and shaved my eyebrows. I was a new person, fake hair, fake eyebrows, fake freckles, new accent and new name. The first few nights were fine with a bit of help. After a rather dodgy deal went wrong, we were on our own. It's amazing how many angels there are in the world and how many people had us stay in their homes. After a long think about how we were going to survive, I decided I would turn Paul's magic skills into a show! We were using rubbish tricks at first, making bits of money busking on the streets. We went all over England earning only £10 a day, the minimum we needed to live on for B & Bs. Sometimes we had enough money to rent places, and other times we would sleep in people's cars or in public toilets.

At Christmas we rented a garage. It was freezing and we found blankets at a local church. We bought a little stove and reused the wax from old candles that had burned out. We had to use a bucket as a toilet and my new diet was fried egg, fried bread, sandwiches, chips and vodka. I needed as much warmth and calories as I could get. I was losing a lot of weight and so was Paul. When there wasn't enough food to go around, Paul would give me half of his.

One time when we were walking along busking in Newquay, a policeman came up to us. I remember my heart beating so fast. At first I was just going to run for it, but my legs wouldn't move. God, was I relieved when all he said was that we were not allowed to busk along that road. For a moment we thought it was all over for us.

There were times when we were doing well and

we had enough money to rent. I even managed to buy some new blue eyes and Paul got a wig. Not long ago I found some old council tax bills that I had kept from a flat we had in Blackpool in our fake names, Cassey and Carl King, which was funny. I learned a lot over that year and a half. I learned that there are so many great people in the world and that you don't need money to have a good life.

Reading this back I can see that many people would see it as very romantic. Running off with your teacher, the whole nation looking out for you and only love and luck to keep you going. But let me tell you, we had our fair share of scary moments. We were chased by two men with an axe one night and met loads of crazy people. There were times when we didn't eat for days and times when we were so cold that we could hardly move.

It wasn't even about sex, which a lot of people insinuated when we first went away. We didn't make love until I was 16. I had spent ages trying to persuade Paul, but he is such a romantic and insisted he wanted to wait, as he wanted it to be special. It was very special; it was my 16th birthday, in Newquay. We had candles and lots of love.

We managed to stay on the run for 18 months. Then we had to face all the stress when we returned from being on the run. We went straight to Portsmouth Crown Court armed with solicitors. After a rather tense battle, Paul was sentenced to 18 months in prison. He served seven months inside, followed by two months on tag.

Naturally, I waited for Paul and we are still very happy together and plan to get married very soon.

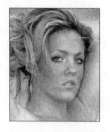

JESSIKA LEZARD

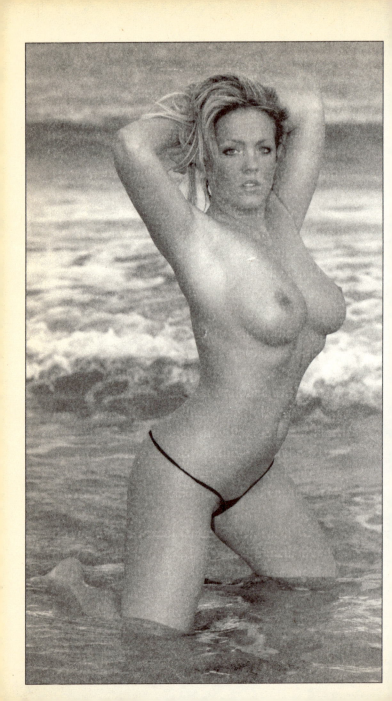

JESSIKA LEZARD

Name: Jessika Lezard
Model/Dance Name: Jessika Lezard
Star Sign: Taurus
Age: 18
Vital Stats: 34E-28-34
Lives: East London
Fave Food: Macdonalds
Fave Drink: Pink Champagne

Where do you work?
I am a full-time glamour model in the UK. However, I have had photos printed in the USA and Europe for an American magazine called *Photogenic*. But apart from that, all my work is in the UK.

How did you get into modelling?
I have done just about every job going, but

until I got into modelling I was never really happy!

I had a very good education and always attended private schools, the last being St Bedes Boarding School in Eastbourne. The problem with private schools is you tend to get pushed into a certain lifestyle. It is expected that you go to University and that you opt for a 'normal' stable career. I found the option of heading in this direction daunting, not to mention boring. Luckily I am a strong character, with lots of drive and had no intention of being bullied into that kind of life.

One day I heard about a job working for Earshot Radio Productions on a new radio station called Arriva, which was due to launch in Brighton. The thought of working in radio really excited me. It was much more of a 'me' career. I knew that, if I sent an application form in saying I was 17 and didn't have any experience, I wouldn't even get to interview stage.

In the end my application form read very well – how could they not give me the job? I had a degree and everything!

On the day of the interview I was really nervous, but, once I was in the room with them, I relaxed and started enjoying it. The interview was going really well, but at the back of my mind the guilt was creeping in about all the lies I had told them to get here.

'OK, guys, I'm sorry. My application form is bullshit. I lied because I wanted to do this so badly.' Everyone was silent, so I continued. 'I'm only 17, but I think I can really do this job well.' You can imagine my relief when they all fell about laughing and told me that I was exactly what they were looking for – someone with a bit of get up and go and enough passion to want to do this that they would go to any extreme. So there I was, breakfast presenter for Arriva FM.

I loved working in radio. I knew my way around the mixing desk and I was involved with producing some shows and worked on editing my own features. I was gutted when after nearly 18 months the station ran out of money and we had to cease broadcasting.

I was now 18 and couldn't face working in a 9–5 job. Lots of people had suggested doing glamour modelling, so I phoned a local photographer and booked a shoot. The pictures turned out OK and I began sending them to various modelling agencies, as well as posting them to online modelling agencies. One day a photographer called Alan Strutt contacted me and asked me to go for a test shoot for the *Sun*. It all went from there.

What's the biggest fee/tip you have ever earned?
£7,000 for a story that appeared in the *Sunday*

People. It was a Kiss 'n' Tell, which was a sex story based on my relationship with Joe Swash (Mickey from *Eastenders*). I was only with Joe on-and-off for about four months and now I regret having done the story.

What highstreet publications have you been in?
After I had done the Kiss 'n' Tell on Joe, I got myself a good PR agent, Craig Johnson, from Unleashed PR. He made sure that I got my face known and it has resulted in me having been seen in most national newspapers, such as the *Daily Star*, the *Sport*, *News of the World*, *Sunday People* and the *Mirror*. You may also of seen me in various lad mags and typical middle-shelf stuff, such as *Heat* etc. I was also voted *Men and Motors* number-one up-and-coming babe in November 2004. Thanks, Craig.

What other work have you done?
Apart from my radio experience, I am also a qualified beauty therapist, having trained at Brighton City College to qualify. I also did a bit of PR work for nightclubs around the West End of London organising club nights.

Do you have any famous friends?
I know lots of famous people, such Dan, Becky,

Ahmed, Emma, all from *Big Brother 5*, Dean Gaffney, Callum Best, Joe Swash (a bit more than most!), Emma Jones, Natalie Denning, Emma Davies, Ashley Cole, Jermain Penant, Ant Scott Lee, Alica Douvell, Andy Newton, and Lee Ray Pakstani

I remember one time I had been to the Cheeky Girls party, which was to celebrate the launch of their single. It was at Capiche nightclub. I went with Jamie and Glen, from the band Pop. In our crowd were Becky and Ahmed from *BB*, Dan Haley *Evetts* from Pop idol and, of course, Craig, my PR agent.

The Cheeky Girls were performing, while we took advantage of the free bar – we were hammered by the time it ended. When the party finished and we got outside, there were hordes of paparazzi, so we were doing a bit of performance for them, which took the form of various lesbian stunts with Becky. It started when we saw a moped parked up outside the club and Becky and me got on and did sexy poses for the papz.

Because we were so drunk we thought that it would be a good idea to jump on a rickshaw to take us to the Embassy nightclub. It was so funny, the paparazzi followed us, jumping up on the rickshaw, while we played to the cameras.

We finally got to the Embassy to top up our

alcohol intake, and we met up with Lisa Scott Lee's designer, Scott Henshaw, whose birthday party it was. Someone was taking pictures of us all and we thought it was for the club's website so were happy to pose. However, I got a call a short while after saying that there was a picture of me licking Ahmed's face on the scandal pages of *Heat* magazine.

What does your family think of the work you do?

When I first started modeling, I didn't tell them. Not because I didn't think they would approve, but because I just wanted to test the water first, to see if it's what I really wanted to do. The unfortunate thing was that I didn't get to tell them at all, as they found out through the media. One day they saw a picture of Joe and me in one of the nationals and it referred to me as his girlfriend, the glamour model.

I guess it's not any parent's ideal job for their child, but they have learned that nothing they can say will stop me from doing what I want to do. My dad is very supportive and just wants to know that I am safe.

My sister loves what I do. She is only 13 and my success has lead to her being very popular with a lot of the boys in the area. One day I opened the door and there were about 15 13-

year-old lads, waving pictures of me asking me to sign them for them – bless! Although they were not so innocent, because not long after that I caught some of them trying to peer through the window while I was getting changed.

My little sis is always ringing me up and asking who I'm out with. One night we were in a club and Lemar was there. I know my little sis loves him, so I rang her and got Lemar to have a chat with her. She still talks about it to this day.

What's your funniest moment?
I had been to the aftershow party for the Television Awards, which was at Funky Buddha in October 2004. I was with two other glamour models and we had had such a good time. We were really pissed and had teamed up with two famous actors. I won't say who they were because I know for a fact that they both had girlfriends. They invited us back to the Grosvenor Hotel for more drinks and we all agreed that we would go.

When we pulled up outside, the guys said that they would go in first and then we should follow them a few minutes later. However, we were all dying for a piss and couldn't wait, so we decided to have a pee right there. So there we were, three glamour models with our knickers around our ankles pissing on the kerb outside the Grosvenor Hotel ... classy, eh?

What's your scariest moment?

The scariest moment I have ever had was feeling out of control with a photographer. He was a very reputable photographer and I was still very inexperienced. He kept pressuring me into doing top-shelf stuff. He told me that this was the only way to get famous and make money. He was really pushy and got a bit angry when I refused.

I am a very confident person and I know exactly what my modelling standards are, so I kept strong and refused to do it. He really took advantage of his position. I saw the horrible side of this business in that shoot: things that that I had been warned about, but I wouldn't have expected it from a reputable photographer. Now I have been in the industry for a while, I know that I am not the only one he has tried this on with. A lot of girls have said the same to me about him.

I can see how ambitious girls are forced into top-shelf magazines and porn. The experience upset me so much that it made me think twice about continuing in this industry. But I decided to use it as a positive experience and learned from it. I was one of the lucky ones.

JESSIKA LEZARD

Have you ever turned down work and why?
I have turned down a lot of website work because you don't have any control as to where the pictures end up! Also, I turn down work with a certain photographer for a tabloid newspaper, because he has such a bad reputation for taking advantage of girls and ripping them off. In fact, every girl that I know who has worked with him has been ripped off and used by him!

Do you have a sexual fantasy?
To be honest, I have done pretty much everything I have wanted to do! But my ultimate fantasy I suppose would be sex with a stranger. He would have to be a complete stranger and I wouldn't even know his name … I would love to live it but I'd need a few drinks first!!! But,then again, I don't know if I would have the guts to go through it.

What's your most memorable sexual encounter?
I was 17 and I had been out all night with my best mate at the time. We had a few too many drinks and we were both flirting around teasing men like most girls do! We got back to her house and we were quite merry. One thing led to another and, before we knew it, we were having sex. It was never anything I had ever thought about doing before. It just happened. However, I did enjoy it

and would probably do it again. We have never spoken about it to this day.

What do you think about group sex? Have you tried it?
I am a very sexual person and would be open to most things. I have had sex with another girl with a man involved but never more than three people. I would probably be up for it though. I think that it's important to give everything a try once, as long as your comfortable with it, then just go for it!

What advice would you give to someone who wanted to get into this business?
There are a few tips I can give. The first is to listen to girls who have made the mistakes and learn by them. If they say to stay away from particular photographers or agents within the business, then stay away. It's easy to think they are saying it because they are jealous and don't want you to do well, but it's not. They, like myself, have learned the hard way and are only protecting you from ending up in a similar situation.

Next tip is, don't take everyone at face value. There are a lot of people that will take advantage of a girl's dreams and ambitions and use it to their advantage.

It helps to try and surround yourself with good friends in this business. You have to associate yourself with a lot of people, because they can help your career. Everyone uses each other to help themselves so it's vital that you keep a group of people around you who you know you can trust.

Finally, have a good and varied portfolio – this is vital in order to sell yourself.

Which bloke do you fancy the most?
Got to say Joe Swash – just to wind him up!!

Tell me a secret ... Well, my biggest secret is a pretty big whopper. I have managed to be 'involved' with half a Premiership Football Team without any of them knowing about each other!

It started one Tuesday night and I was working in a bar, called the Event, in Brighton. I had only been working there for about two months and got the job after breaking up from my long-term boyfriend. I had been with my boyfriend for two-and-a-half years and working in a bar was a great way to meet new people.

The night was pretty quiet until a group of footballers coming in. They had been on a night out and were full of high spirits. It was great because they really cheered me up. They were drinking vodka and, every time they ordered a single, I was giving them all triples. By the end of the night they were all pretty wasted. Not content with stopping when last orders were called, they talked about going back to one of the players' houses, who lived in Brighton, for more booze.

They invited me back with them and waited until I had finished work. I was only in my work clothes, but I had been having such a laugh with them, I thought Why not? Even though I was the only girl, it didn't matter. Most of my mates are guys and they just thought of me as 'one of the lads'.

We got back to the apartment, which was lovely, and continued with the banter. Some started playing computer games and the others were playing pool. The guys were very flirtatious and through the evening one by one came up to me and asked me for my number. I gave it to them, not really thinking too much of it. I left on my own and got a cab home.

What happened next was really bizarre. Over the next two weeks all six players who I had given my number to were texting non-stop. I had told each one not to tell anyone about the contact and all had agreed. I remember sitting with my friends thinking of what to text them and then sending them all the same message and we sat around all laughing and they all replied simultaneously. The messages they were texting to me ranged from 'MAKES A CHANGE TO MEET A NICE GIRL, I'M GLAD I MET YOU x' to 'I WANT KISS EVERY INCH OF YOUR BODY AND THEN ...' etc.

There was one player that I did like and actually took him up on his offer for a night out. He picked me up and we went to Brighton to the cinema to watch *Pay Cheque*. It was funny really because he didn't really understand the film and I had to continuously explain it to him.

I had said to this guy that I thought it was best if he didn't tell anyone, even his co-players, that we had been out together. He seemed happy about this, as most girls he had been with wanted the glory of being with a footie player.

He rang me one day when they were all on a coach travelling to a match. He was having a laugh with me and jokingly asked if I fancied a foursome. I told him that wasn't going to happen and that he knew who my favourite was. The guy on the phone started relaying my message, obviously assuming it was he who was my favourite. Within minutes, my phone was going mad, with text message after text message from all the players, each saying that they knew secretly it was them that was my fave. I had to laugh.

I kept the texting going for a bit longer, as I was

enjoying playing with them all. It was good entertainment. My ex-boyfriend was also a football player and actually played for a rival team. One day they were playing each other and I couldn't resist, so I went along to watch. During the game, one of the players commented to my ex about the fact that I was seeing someone from the rival team. A fight broke out on the pitch.

After the match the manager approached me in the players' lounge and told me that I should stay away from his boys and not come to any more football matches. I didn't go back to watch any more football, but I didn't stay away from the boys!

After a while I got a bit bored with the games and I was getting very busy with my modelling, so I fizzled the texting out. I do still laugh to myself sometimes. I can't believe that they are so sure of themselves that they would never dream of a woman playing them. It's usually them that boast about their conquests. But I played them all and made them all believe they were special. Come on, if men can do it, why can't we!!

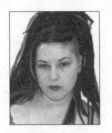

ALEXANDRA

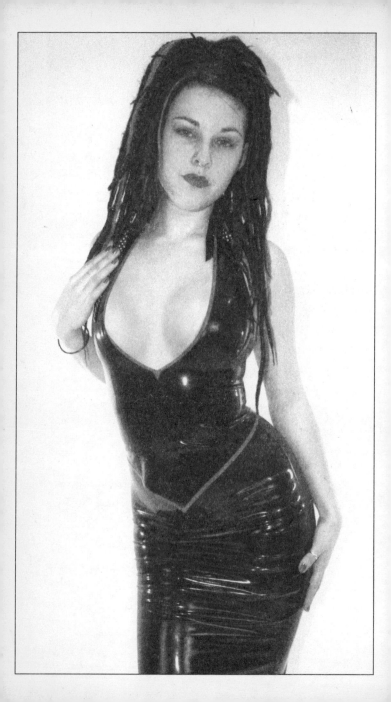

ALEXANDRA

Name: Alexandra Parsons
Model/Dance Name: Alexandra
Star Sign: Scorpio
Age: 20
Vital Stats: 34D-27-37
Lives: Stoke Newington, London
Fave Food: Sushi
Fave Drink: Gin & tonic

Where do you work?

I do fetish, alternative and glamour work country-wide as well as internationally, although I'm London based.

I recently worked with a guy who does a lot of shoots for the fetish magazines *Skin Two* and *Marquis*. I don't know if my pictures will be published there, as they pick a few from his portfolio every month or so. His photography demands quite a lot from the model – he doesn't believe models are subject to everyday concerns, such as gravity, so it was straining, but the results were good.

I did a job in Rotherham, which is a small Yorkshire town, to do some femdom work for a couple who run a few paysites. They have a really cute enterprise – while the kids are out at school, they invite models round for shoots. Their kids have no idea that the garage that they aren't allowed in is actually a perfect 50s schoolroom replica (plus lots of whips etc on the walls)

I also did a job in Zurich. I went with my partner to do a shoot with a guy who lived in the middle of nowhere. The house was an old restaurant, so very large. I was just doing the usual glamour portfolio-style work, but in such a strange context. At night we got so freaked out we locked the door to our room and peed in the sink because we were too afraid to walk down the hall!

How did you get into modelling?

I started off by doing gothic fashion modelling with a lovely Canadian photographer, Stephane Lord, when I was 16. He contacted me through a gothic website where lots of people put their details on. It's a useful tool. Anyway, his job required me to wander round the industrial wasteland of King's

ALEXANDRA

Cross finding interesting textures in the brickwork to pose against! I still rate the photographs he first took of me as amongst my best – they've been published in a couple of German magazines!

This first job really gave me a taste for modelling and made me consider for the first time whether this was something I wanted to do. I never really thought I could make it as a model, because I wasn't tall enough and was too large (not a size 6 and not 6 foot tall!). Working in a niche market, as I do, means that I can get away with a lot more.

After this first job, I didn't really move towards the glamour industry for a while. I was underage, therefore waited until my 18th birthday to take things further. I realised that most of the money is to be made in the glamour-and-nude modelling industry, therefore, I thought I'd give it a shot. My first nude work was actually doing the nude exhibit thing in Selfridges for Spencer Tunick. The pictures were all in the papers and it was wonderful fun. It's so liberating being naked somewhere where you normally go to buy your make-up! That sense of liberation, of breaking taboos, is perhaps what's kept me interested.

What's the biggest fee/tip you have ever earned?

The best thing I've ever done was work for this one guy who wanted me to come to his apartment in South Kensington. I was a bit apprehensive, because I don't really hold with going to clients' houses, but it was a lovely place. Basically, he wanted to film me kicking bottles for two hours (for £80ph – not bad). I had to teeter about in a rubber dress and stilettos kicking these two-litre Evian bottles that were full of water. They were suspended from the ceiling from string. It was hilarious, because it was so difficult to keep upright. I don't know how I managed to drag it out to two hours though – it was very tedious! Well that's the most bizarre thing I've ever been asked to do anyway. God knows what he does with the video – I don't want to think about that really, do I?

What highstreet publications have you been in?

I haven't been in any publications yet but have recently become a Suicide Girl (www.suicidegirls.com), which I guess is high profile. Nearly everyone I know knows about this site (alternative girls getting naked!). This involves you sending off a set of what they consider to be original images and then hopefully getting chosen. I worked with a guy who I'd worked for before who, to be honest, didn't do as good a job as I'd hoped! I now feel annoyed I didn't get pictures up there that I was happier with – and lots of my

ALEXANDRA

friends and acquaintances see them. I can always send more off though, so it's not really a problem.

Other than that, I've had pictures of me exhibited at the Erotica trade show. Also I worked at the London Edge Trade Show a couple of times etc, as well as with one guy, Ron Chapple, who does gorgeous stock images in Hawaii. His images are really clean, fashiony, but taking a new approach. He does a lot of wide-angled-lens work, which is always flattering and kooky.

What other work have you done?

I model part-time in order to fund my academic career. I am currently an English Literature student on one of the most prestigious courses in the country. It's very interesting, but demanding. It's peculiar to go to Uni with one set of friends who have no idea about my other life! They all have bar jobs or rich mummies and daddies to get them through the next few years – I do something much more entertaining and consequently have lots more money to play with!

My course is very varied. I have been reading St Augustine's *Confessions* (who would have thought this traditionally Christian man was initially such a cad!) and Swift's *Gulliver's Travels* – which is anything but a children's book. I have read a lot of Greek tragedy and epics – which form the background to much of Western thought and literary tradition.

I always feel slightly odd about juxtaposing an academically rigorous course with the stereotypically air-headed job of being a model! It's always fun telling people who think you're just slacking/stupid what you do the rest of the time.

I have just finished doing a job where I wrote CVs for unemployed people. This was also a part-time job alongside my studies and was very interesting. Coming from a rather privileged background, I have never previously met anyone who'd completely failed their GCSEs. It was an eye-opener and got me thinking about a totally different kind of life.

I have also just finished a foundation art course at Central Saint Martin's School of Art. It was fun, but tiring as I had to work so many hours to fund it. Self-discipline was hard.

Do you have any famous friends?
I guess my most famous friend is Morrigan Hel.

What does your family think of the work you do?
My family don't really know fully what it is that I do. My immediate family have known I've done fashion modelling for a while, but don't really have any opinion on that.

ALEXANDRA

Although … it was my 20th birthday recently. I was out for dinner with my family to celebrate this at my favourite Indian in Dulwich, London. Just before we started eating, my father commented that he'd seen my site! Now, I've never told him I had a site and was quite shocked. It's not so much that he's seen it (although who wants their father looking at them naked) but that he mentioned it. Why couldn't he be more English about it and not bring it up? Anyway, he doesn't mind – he thinks I'm an enterprising young lady. And I guess he's right about that!

What's your funniest moment?

I was in a Wetherspoons pub with my boyfriend and a few others for a cheap and raucous Friday night. The night was going well as always (as one would expect with £5 pitchers on offer) when I somehow, in a fuzzy drunken state, got tricked into starting a conversation with a red-faced, Scottish football-shirted hooligan. He recognised me from modelling somewhere or other, but through the haze I can't remember where.

Anyway, I didn't manage to extricate myself from this situation at all and everyone else found it really rather funny. This carried on for a bit, until he sent me down to the bar to get us both a drink. The foolish, foolish man gave me a twenty-pound note. I returned victorious with about eight Goldschlagers for me and all my friends and no change for him whatsoever. He started getting really shirty with me, which I dealt with by accidentally drinking nearly all of these shooters myself. Through the fog, I managed to make out the hooligan: 'Ah reeealy woant tae huv seeeax, you ken whut ah mean, jist a wee f*** that's all.'

It turned out that, because of the drinks incident, he felt he was due some recompense for his troubles and was trying to convince my boyfriend to let him drag me off into the toilets for a quick one. It was so funny – he reassured us with how quick he would be, as though the only problem with his request would be time away from my night out! When we finally convinced him it really wasn't going to happen, he tried the same tactics with every other female in the group. This all happened at the same time that his only slightly more reasonable French friend was being fended off by us summoning the full extent of our French GCSE language skills to tell him that we were hot swimming pools, that we lived in a fishing lake, our green door had a headache and that his mother was a guinea pig ... Perhaps I should of continued studying my French to an advanced level!

ALEXANDRA

What's your scariest moment?

Paranoia induced by the house in Zurich! Other than that, I do fetish work a lot of the time, including play-piercing work. I was working in Reading, at F1 Studios with a guy wanting to get interesting things in his portfolio. I was doing piercing, as I have been doing for years, when all of a sudden one hurt way more than it was meant to. I looked down and saw that one was bleeding on my stomach, which never normally happens. I took it out, trying to pretend that nothing was wrong so as not to look unprofessional, and the thing started bleeding just below my skin. This resulted in a large patch (about as big as the base of a mug) of purple bruising which was blood floating around under the skin. I resolved to be more careful in the future.

Have you ever turned down work and why?

Yes. I was asked to work with a guy just doing portfolio glamour, fashion, bit of nude. We agreed rates, studio, date and time. I was all set, until the day before, when he decided that actually what he wanted was to be buggered by a mistress with a strap-on! I was so annoyed because it was so deceitful of him not to say this straight off. Now, as a professional model I'm clearly not interested in this kind of thing. It pissed me off because he obviously thought that, because we'd got this far, I'd be more up for just going along with what he wanted. Men!

Do you have a sexual fantasy?

There's this beautiful blonde girl I know who wears a lot of military uniforms and has a great cleavage. She's not a close friend, but closer than an acquaintance. She always looks immaculate in a German kind of a way. My fantasy is that we're at a party and I push her up the stairs and into a random room. She's not too sure what's going on, but doesn't mind either. I tie her up and force her to have sex with me. I'm not sure how, as this is a recent fantasy so many variables change each time.

What's your most memorable sexual encounter?

When I was much younger I used to go out with a tall blond transvestite. He was loads of fun. Once we drove into the middle of nowhere and spied upon a church in the middle of a small village green in Berkshire. We saw a couple of people coming out, so knew it was open. We went in and it all seemed very quiet. It was a lovely place – very medieval. We didn't dare disturb the flower arrangement on the altar – but we had rather loud and inappropriate sex in one of the alcoves. Just as we finished, some rather surprised people came in!

ALEXANDRA

What do you think about group sex? Have you tried it?

I haven't tried it, but mainly through lack of opportunity. I wouldn't not try it – it sounds like a laugh, but at the moment I'm in a long-term relationship so can't play around with things like that. My boyfriend has, though. He'd got back to one of his friends' houses and, inevitably, all the clothes started flying off. Everybody was so wasted anyway, I don't think anyone is in a position to regret it – it was all in good fun. I just find it funny that so many of my friends have fooled around then forgotten about it! I don't know anyone who regrets it – which encourages me all the more!

What advice would you give to someone who wanted to get into this business?

That it's hard work and reputation is everything! If you aren't going to bother replying to emails and chasing things up, you won't get anywhere. I am always a bit reticent about passing on my contacts to friends, because often they don't realise you can't mess around with studio bookings. I always turn up on time and ready – I don't understand why a lot of models don't, as it gives the rest of us a hard time!

TELL ME A SECRET

Which bloke do you fancy the most?
Nick Cave! He's not handsome in a traditional sense, but his strange looks are somehow appealing!

Tell me a secret ... I was 15 and bored. I wandered into the basement of a Soho café and sat down expectantly. After a while, I got talking to a man in his mid-30s about paganism, *Skin Two* magazine, learning French and God knows what else. We got on surprisingly well: next thing we knew it was five hours later and we'd already kissed. He seemed so exciting to me: he had a shaved head, a motorbike, listened to rock music and went to fetish clubs.

I didn't tell him how old I was. I lied and said I was 18 and he bought it. He still thought that was terribly young, but what can I say? It seemed like a good idea (to both of us) at the time. Things progressed slowly but surely. We met up about once a week and went to a movie, or out for a meal. It wasn't particularly intense, so I was somewhat surprised that he viewed me as his one most important partner. I guess he was important to me too: this was my first serious relationship and the first person that made me realise I wasn't some kind of hideous troll!

It was all rather cute and romantic, even if from

the outside it seems wrong and incomprehensible. I felt so sorry for my poor mother. I didn't have a very good relationship with my parents, and things were always rather tense at home. They arranged a family holiday to some small town in the middle of France and I couldn't imagine anything worse. I told them this and asked them not to book it for me, but they did. On the morning we were due to go, I pretended to go out to post a letter. At the bottom of the road, this boyfriend was waiting for me on his motorbike and we jetted off and away from there. In retrospect, that does seem really selfish and a terribly teenage thing to do: oh well! We spent the day eating lots, doing rude things and then went to the theatre. Quite civilised, really.

Things started to change after a few months and until now I have not shared the details of my relationship with anyone. We trusted each other more, had unlimited picnics in the middle of nowhere together and were pretty certain that this was working out nicely. He had a fantastically strong and magnetic character: I really wanted to give all of me to him. He had always wanted to try out a 24/7 dominant-submissive relationship, so, rather than just role-play in the bedroom, we gave it a go. I spent hours poring over the cuter, text-based BDSM websites, wondering what it would be like. I learned all about collaring (the submissive partner wears a token of their obedience at all times, either a collar or some form of necklace), Japanese tea ceremonies and so on. How did this feed into our relationship? It seemed mainly to involve tedious things such as always being the one to fetch the coffee, agree to whatever he wanted and so on. We were both learning and didn't yet know what worked for us. It's all very well playing around with bondage and obedience in the bedroom, but it didn't transfer very well for us in real life.

I became bitter about this state of affairs, but, like the 15-year-old I was, didn't talk reasonably about my issues with this. I felt like our relationship could never go back to how it was before and I'd be damned if I'd do anything more for someone else. The relationship broke down because I decided I didn't want to play any more and we didn't discuss things properly. I was young and enthusiastic about meeting new boys.

How has this affected my life? Well, we're still nominally friends. I see him about once a year, and we go out for dinner and still get on really well. We don't fit into each other's life though: he has his friends and I have mine. He has left one legacy though – the interest in fetish practices.

While I don't understand people who only have one fetish and can only enjoy sex if that one thing happens, I do enjoy a bit of variety. I followed up my dominant biker boyfriend with a somewhat younger transvestite. He was insecure, tall, loved pink, industrial music and exhibitionism. We had all the fun, but it was lots of hassle too; sorting out other people's issues all the time isn't great entertainment.

One day we were shopping in a little fetish and bondage shop for cute spikey shoes. The woman who worked there asked me if I wanted a part-time job and I said yes. I worked in the fetish shop for about a year. We sold sex toys, but it was mainly bondage gear and rubber clothing. Aside from providing entertainment and being rather more a social occasion than a job (customers always stayed for cups of tea), it allowed me to get 50% off rubber, corsetry and PVC clothing. I went mad buying all these beautiful clothes to wear to fetish clubs. It was great.

The main points of interest in working in this shop were the customers. We (naturally) got some fantastically peculiar people in. There was one man who always ordered complicated restraints. He always wanted to test them out while in the shop and we didn't really mind too much. His thing (so it seemed) was trying to get out of these damned things whilst someone watched. Of course, we couldn't let him see us watching him as that would have been bad and wrong, so we went downstairs (to his great frustration) and watched him on CCTV. There was nothing funnier than watching a middle-aged man writhe around on a shop floor and like it! We also had another man in who would always stare longingly at our wigs and shoes. Our shoes went up to a size 12 – they were *meant* for men! But he'd always insisted that actually that size-10 pair of red patent stilettos was for his wife/friend. So silly though – who buys wigs and shoes for their wives?

The most worrying of all our clientele was a rather nervous but pleasant man who came in without fail every single Saturday afternoon to buy pairs of see-through, baby-blue plastic pants. Ewww ... We couldn't work out what he did with them to need a new pair every single week – or whether he just liked the thrill of buying them! Weird ... But it was loads of fun. I stopped working there when exam pressure built up, but I wish I hadn't: I loved it there! It's just always a challenge to know what to say about it on your CV ...

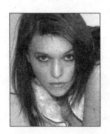

ELLIE

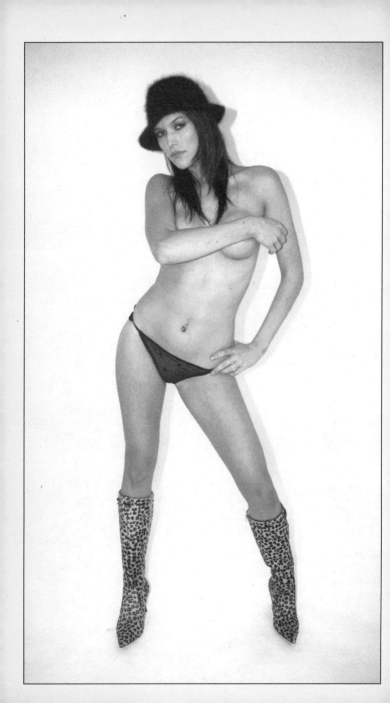

ELLIE

Name: Eleanor Faye Hutchinson
Model/Dance Name: Ellie
Star Sign: Scorpio
Age: 22
Vital Stats: 34C-26-33
Lives: York
Fave Food: Greek salads, shell fish, marmite on cold toast
Fave Drink: Dry white wine, full-sugar Coke

Where do you work?

I am a full-time student at Manchester Met Uni and currently coming to the end of a three-year degree in media. I do part-time modelling to earn a bit of extra cash as an aid to funding my education.

I have been trying to break into the modelling world for a few years now. Throughout the duration of my short career in the modelling field, I have become more certain that this is a career I would love to pursue.

My first-ever modelling job came only two years ago in 'The Girls of Manchester Universities Calendar'. I was Miss February and posed naked and covered in the rose petals (AKA *American Beauty*) stance. Afterwards an agency in Manchester head-hunted me and I joined their books.

Since I have been modelling, I have discovered how difficult it really is to break into a commercial market. My jobs to date have included a fashion spread for the *Daily Mail* newspaper; a catalogue shoot for the Jonathan Seagull Catalogue Dickens International Ltd; a sporting clothes shoot for photographer Mike Gallaway internet photograph center; a nightwear photo shoot for Refinery, Manchester; a television advertisement for Adidas Predator Football boots; a television advertisement for GHD Hair straightness; catwalk fashion shows for York Technical College Fashion department end of year show July 2002; July 2003 Catwalk Fashion show for Cancer Research, High Society nightclub Liverpool, sponsored by Base Clothing, Ravel Shoes and Adidas.

In February 2004 I did the Netto in-store clothing advertisements and photographs used

ELLIE

for packaging; a television advertisement for *Ministry Of Sound – Big Tunes* Album; a catalogue shoot for the Additions spring/summer catalogue: home furnishing sofa collection. I guess it sounds a lot when you say it all in one go, but over two years it's not what I would class as regular work.

I also do a bit of model promo work. This work includes things such as being a regular Red Square promo girl for Key 103, Manchester-based radio station. Also, through the company Keystone, I do promo jobs for Boots, Kodak, Esure Insurance. Most recently I have been doing in-store promo modelling for the Diesel clothing store in King Street, Manchester.

Last but not least I also do TV presenting on local TV Channel, York TV.

How did you get into modelling?

I was spotted in the street in my first year of Uni at the age of 20 by two guys putting together a 'Girls of Manchester Universities Calendar'. I was living in Manchester at the time, so I went to the casting and got chosen for it. Afterwards I was approached by another girl, who was in the calendar and who scouted for her agency in Manchester. I went along to the agency and they put me on their books. Afterwards I got some test shots done but as a student it's difficult to continually refresh your portfolio with new pictures as they cost so much money, and as my appearance has changed in the last two years I find it difficult for my book to keep up with my face.

As previously mentioned I feel that I haven't received my big break as yet! I am desperate to make an impression and believe I have the look, talent and personality to make a good impression on the glamour-modelling world. I certainly feel that I have paid my dues in crappy menial jobs, which pay dick and leave you feeling like a fool for even having the dream of wanting to pursue this career. However, unlike some, I have never let this dampen my spirits (although I feel like my bonfire has almost been well and truly pissed out enough times) and I will work my damn hardest until something comes my way, even if I die trying.

What's the biggest fee/tip you have ever earned?

My wish one day is to be paid thousands for a shoot abroad with loads of free extras; right now my biggest payment to date is the £450 I received from the Ministry Of Sound TV commercial.

What other work have you done?

After finishing at Grey Coat Hospital School, Westminster, London, I moved to York and did

ELLIE

my final two years at Fulford School in York. I gained nine GCSEs and three A levels. I figured after that I didn't want to go straight to university. So I took four months out and went travelling around Australia. Then in 2002 I started Manchester University, where I'm doing a degree in Film and Media Studies.

Obviously, as a student, I need to earn money. I don't earn enough from my modelling yet to keep me going. I have done lots of jobs from working in a bakery and Pizza Hut, to telecommunications and bars.

In between uni, model assignments and part-time work, I also keep auditioning and did manage to get to the final ten in the nationwide MTV Presenter search 2004.

What highstreet publications have you been in?
Mainly catalogues etc and I have been in the *Daily Mail*.

Do you have any famous friends?
One day it will be me who is the famous name being used in a book such as this and I say bloody well use it because if I had ever met anybody famous I would definitely be name-dropping right now ... unfortunately I haven't.

TELL ME A SECRET

What does your family think of the work you do?
My parents are supportive of my choices, although university was packed into the deal of my chosen line of work. Education in my parents' eyes is essential whatever career path I decide to take. My father, however, was not over the moon about my pursuit of modelling. I think he believed it interfered with my education. I'm still doing it despite his reservations. He told me never to get a tattoo – I did (two) and never to get any piercings – I did (ears, belly button, tongue). I do respect him but I will always follow my heart and own wishes.

What's your funniest moment?
Me and my female friend got really f***ed one night and decided to have a bath together when we got home. We had a snog and fumble etc. But the funniest part about it was that we were running around the house starkers, slipping all over the floor and banging into everything because we were totally wet. When we woke up the next day we had bruises everywhere. It looked like we had both had a right battering. Although we learned a good lesson: never do drunken, naked running when wet, particularly on laminate flooring. And now we are much more sexually wise. Very funny and, thank God, we are

ELLIE

still friends today, despite the random craziness of the experience!

What's your scariest moment?

My scariest moment would have to be when I was in Australia travelling with my friend Tessa. We were in the last leg of our trip travelling up the east coast of Australia and had reached Cairns.

In Cairns, me, Tessa and two friends of ours went on the hunt for some weed, so we could have a joint later on the beach. We were told by some other travellers to go to the promenade, near the beach and ask any of the people sat on the picnic tables. We did this and an old hippy-looking white guy said he'd sort us out. He directed us on to an aborigine lady, who said we had to follow her 'cause the police were watching.

Being four stupid 19-year-olds, we did. She walked up the road and kept on walking out of the town. I don't know why we followed, but we thought we'd come this far and we really needed a joint, so we followed some more.

It started to get scary when we found ourselves walking through a multi-storey car park into a ghetto-like area of houses. At this point we all wanted to go, but she said we were there now. So we waited at this house, until a huge black guy, over six foot and really wide, came out of a doorway of the house. He asked us to show our money. We were all really scared so we asked for the weed. He handed over this tiny bag with a few crumbs of green in it and then said, '$50'. We were all too scared to argue, as two more guys appeared from behind him. We gave him the money and walked away sharpish. We knew someone was following us for a while up to the car park, so when we got there we just ran back into the town.

It was such a stupid thing to have done. Anything could have happened! But it taught me to always be wary and cautious of anyone you meet for the first time.

Have you ever turned down work and why?

A model friend of mine put me in touch with an independent photographer in order to earn some extra money. I wasn't being put forward for many castings with my agency, so agreed to do this.

It's not really allowed and frowned upon by the agency, but I needed the money. Anyway, the photographer I worked for in Manchester began turning up at the local shop I worked at, which also happened to be next door to my house. He was claiming he was in the area for one reason or another: haircuts, laundry etc. I thought this was pretty unlikely, as I lived in the scummiest student area of Manchester. He was quite well off and I

ELLIE

couldn't imagine why the hell he was coming to this district for haircuts etc. I did two jobs for him. He was an independent photographer, who sold on his pictures after they had been shot to open websites and magazines. One day he asked me again if I wanted to use his studio. By this time I had become suspicious as he'd visited my shop four times. I felt totally unsafe and uneasy and there was no way I was going to his studio, which was above his home. I made some excuse and then didn't answer his calls.

I don't know if I may have sold myself short, but I didn't want to put myself into any danger and I had to go with my gut feeling. I now only ever do the jobs my legitimate agency organises for me and only attend their castings.

Do you have a sexual fantasy?

My sexual fantasy would be to have sex in the hall of mirrors in the fun fair. It would have to be in a place where me and my boyfriend couldn't be found but our images would be projected on all the mirrors so every oneelse could see (including us). We would be trying out all different positions, watching ourselves do it ... Mmm sexy! Also knowing that other people can see us and are probably God-damn jealous is an even bigger buzz!

TELL ME A SECRET

What's your most memorable sexual encounter?
Boring as it might sound, it was with my boyfriend. We decided to go to a petting zoo and have a picnic etc. It was a really hot day and we got really horny while walking round. There was nowhere private we could sneak into, as there were kids everywhere. So on the drive back home, my boyfriend did a detour into this well obvious open field.

There was a farmer in the far distance on a tractor, but we did it anyway. My dress hitched up, he lifted me on to the bonnet of his car. It was so good I didn't care if passing cars or the farmer could see us. I just lay back in the sunshine and enjoyed it.

However, when we returned home there was a large dent in the front of his car, which both his parents noticed, but we had to keep straight faces as the damage was looked at. I didn't realise my bum was so big!

What do you think about group sex? Have you tried it?
One on one is the only route for me. I like to be the most important person in the room – always.

What advice would you give to someone who wanted to get into this business?
Prepare yourself for the long haul. You get out of

ELLIE

it what you put into it. Therefore, the more tests you get the better your book will look. The person with the best pictures in the room at a casting – it doesn't matter if you are the best-looking or not – will get the job. Always renew tests and, although that can be expensive, you can get round it by doing tests for free. The more pictures you have, the greater the opportunity to create a better future.

Which bloke do you fancy the most?
Mine!

Tell me a secret ... Since the age of 14 I started to notice that all of the girls around me, friends and my sisters, were developing into women and I was being left behind. All the girls were starting their periods and developing breasts and I remained as tomboyish as ever! It wasn't so bad when I lived in London and went to an all-girls school as I excelled in sports and did a lot of dance, ballet, tap, modern, jazz, and this became my disguise. But when my parents moved us to York, I had to attend a mixed comprehensive. This is where I really started to feel different and unhappy, as the boys' reaction to my lack of development in the chest area evolved into teasing and the girls, I guess, just found it amusing.

It didn't matter how good at dance I was, how many shows I did or how many sports teams I joined, the topic of importance now was boyfriends and I didn't have one. This made me weird to the other girls and made it even more difficult to fit in at a new school!

I began to feel depressed about the situation. I went to my GP but she just laughed and in a highly patronising manner said, 'Oh, you'll grow soon, give it time.' It was so distressing that even my GP found it funny that my mum took me to the family planning clinic at the age of fifteen-and-a-half, so I could be put on the contraceptive pill to kick-start developing something. Thank God for my mum, because at every point my flat chest has been a problem (all the time) for me growing up she has tried her best to support me and try and fix the situation.

As I grew older and went to college, the early taking of the pill did help a little, I suppose, as I had started my periods and grown to – wow – a size 34A! I never had problems getting boyfriends after that, I think, because I became the loud, funny, crazy one always up for getting pissed and making people laugh. I suppose I've never been unhappy with my face, it's quite pretty, so I felt that my face and personality were a positive.

My anxiety about my body continued right up

ELLIE

to the end of my teens and into my twenties, where I remained a size 34A. I would never show my top half to boyfriends even though I had been with them for years and was in two long-term sexual relationships from the age of 16 to 20.

After college I went travelling to Australia at the age of 19, then enrolled in a three-year uni course, always making lots of friends along the way, and everything else in my life was reasonably good and happy. I even met the boyfriend I have now when I hit 20, who has become my best friend and biggest support. However, despite his friendship and love, it never took away my insecurities.

When I moved to Manchester when I first began uni, I was taken on by a modelling agency. But, once again, I felt that my flat chest was hindering me in the career I wished to pursue. I felt that my face and personality gave me the upper hand on most girls at the castings but my body let me down. I therefore came to the decision in August 2004 that I was going to have breast-enlargement surgery. I discussed it with my parents and, although they were unhappy with me getting finance to pay for them, they eventually gave in and supported me as they knew this was something I had always been unhappy about and wanted to change. My boyfriend was also really supportive and was very discreet about the whole thing.

I suppose being with a modelling agency did encourage me slightly more to go for it, but it was not the reason behind my decision. It was something I had to do for myself in order to feel more confident with my body. However, if my career chances improve because of it then the results are better than I could have imagined.

I didn't tell a lot of people about the operation as I didn't want to hear negative opinions about it (I know a lot of people have them) and this was no one else's decision but mine. I wasn't getting it done for anyone but me!

The wait from my first consultation in September 2004 to my actual op in November, although short, to me was agonisingly long! I just wanted it to be done tomorrow and the healing to be over with too! Now they're done, I couldn't be more happy. I am in the process of having my portfolio updated and have received a really positive response from friends, family and my agency who insist this will be a big turning point for me and my career as a model (I hope so anyway). My ambition as a model is to grace the covers and inside spreads of women's magazines and do the sexy stuff for the likes of *FHM* and *Loaded* etc. I feel much more confident and

ELLIE

physically I know I look really good now. Good enough to be up there with the best glamour models around now. I feel like I can take on any challenge that may be in front of me and succeed in a career in modelling, and this is a confidence I never had before.

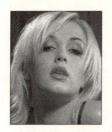

KACIE LOU

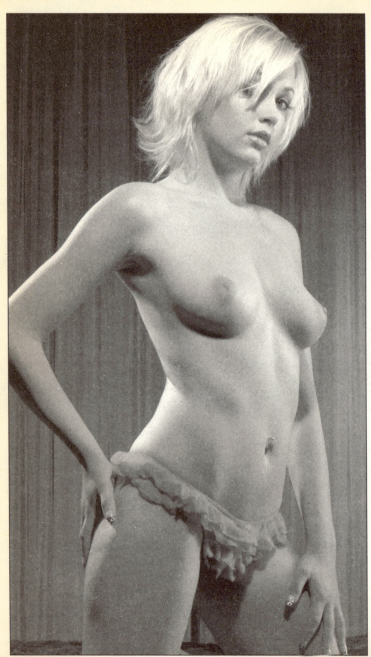

Photo © Martin Levenson

KACIE LOU

Name: Stephanie Harris
Model/Dance Name: Kacie Lou
Star Sign: Gemini
Age: 18
Vital Stats: 36B-26-32
Lives: Milton Keynes
Fave Food: Fillet of beef
Fave Drink: White wine

Where do you work?
I have been modelling for three years now but it has only really started to take off since I turned 18, which was in May 2004. There was a new law that came out, which stated that you had to be 18 to model topless, nude etc, so I couldn't wait until I turned 18 to really kick my career off.

I did have an assignment in Lanzarote in

TELL ME A SECRET

January 2005, which was a week-long shoot involving G/G (Girl/Girl) for an adult channel called TVX. Also I am involved in another project for TVX, which is also another G/G shoot.

I have been in a few lads' magazine, such as *ICE*, which was a feature called 'The girl next door', for their December 2004 edition.

My ambition is to travel the world on assignments. I want to be the next Jordan.

How did you get into modelling?

I was just turning 16 when I was introduced to glamour modelling. My godfather actually introduced me to it. His wife used to be a glamour model and he used to be a photographer. He kept saying to me, 'You could be a glamour model. How about you let me take some pictures of you and see how it goes from there?' So I agreed. I didn't like the photos at all, but still decided to upload them on to a modelling website, which was called Net-Model.

As soon as I uploaded them on to the website and filled in all the details, I was getting emails straight away. I was so excited I thought to myself, I can actually do this.

I was also on a website called faceparty. This wasn't an actual modelling website, just a site where people go and look at other people's profiles and their pictures. A couple of weeks after I had uploaded my images on to faceparty I had an email from a photographer in Milton Keynes, which is where I am based. He owned a studio and was interested in shooting a test, so I went along. It was so nerve-racking but I loved every minute of it.

A couple of weeks after my shoot I had an email from the photographer saying that he was interested in me and wanted to know if I would be interested in working with him for a website. I thought this was a great opportunity, so I agreed to this and we arranged for me to go back to his studio. After a month, the site was up and running and it was called MkBabes, The money wasn't much but I was so excited that I had my own website.

Six months later I decided that I didn't want to be on MkBabes any more and I decided to leave. Since then I have worked with many photographers, professional and amateurs, including: Alan Strutt (Page 3 photographer), Jens Wikholm (Popstar), Cris James, Shaun MacManus, Martin Levenson, Paul West, Dave Davies ... and many more.

While building up my portfolio, I have also been shooting content for my website, which is called KacieLou.com. I am also starting to shoot content for my next website, which is going to be more on the adult side of the industry.

My images have recently been sent to Sky One, soccer AM girls and the *Daily Sport*, so I could have many more projects in the coming months.

What's the biggest fee/tip you have ever earned?
The most amount of money I have been paid for shooting would have to be Hard G/G. I was paid £250 for a three-to-four hour shoot.

What highstreet publications have you been in?
At the moment I have not appeared in any top magazines or newspapers, but I have lots of things lined up at the moment, such as *ICE* Magazine, TVX, Sky One, *Daily Sport*, *Front* and *Zoo* magazine

What other work have you done?
Currently glamour modelling is my part-time job, as I am not yet with an agency. I am due to go and see Samantha Bond's agency in London shortly, as they were interested in seeing me after they saw my images.

My website is going really well and I'm really exciting about developing this side of the business. I have got lots of ideas, particularly with the adult stuff – well they do say that's where the money is.

KACIE LOU

Less exciting is my full-time job, which is office based at a company called Octel. I have been there for about four months now. It is a temporary position, but I am hoping to be kept on after my six months.

Do you have any famous friends?
I haven't got any famous friends at the moment. I know people that know Jordan, Blue, the boys from *Dream Team* etc.

I have also worked with Jordan's best friend, who is a make-up artist. She was the make-up artist for my test shoot, which I did for the *Sun* newspaper last year.

What does your family think of the work you do?
My family has stuck by me ever since I started glamour modelling. My dad was always saying to me that I should be a model. They are the reason I had the guts to give it a try.

My family are proud of me for what I do and I think that's the way it should be. To have friends and family standing by me in this difficult line of career is the most important thing to me.

My parents are just like me; if the modelling front is quiet, they get upset because I am not getting any work and if I get really busy they are really happy for me.

TELL ME A SECRET

What's your funniest moment?

The funniest moment I have ever had was when I was at a photo shoot in Northampton. I was with another model friend of mine, Natalie B, and another friend who was interested in becoming a model. It was a bondage shoot. We were toying with the idea of cancelling the shoot as none of us was particularly into bondage. But we went ahead and got on the train to Northampton. When we reached our destination we decided that we would go and get a few bottles of alcohol just so that the bondage wouldn't hurt so much.

We met the photographer and he took us to his apartment, where we had a few drinks and a laugh. We decided which outfits we were going to wear and the type of bondage it was going to be. It was all involving ropes, chains and gags. We weren't too keen on the gags, but we agreed to go ahead with it.

I was the first model to pose. The photographer decided that we were going to shoot some solo sets and also duo sets. I got ready and the photographer got me tied up. This part was OK, as I was the only model shooting that set so there was nothing to pull on my arms and legs.

We finished the solo sets and started on the duo sets. It was so funny by this time, as we had been at the shoot for three hours and were quite drunk. The photographer tied Natalie and me together, which was quite painful. We were drunk and kept moving about, which was making the ropes tighter.

At last, we got to the last set, which was in the bath. The bath was tiny so it was quite difficult to move around, especially as there were two models in the bath tied up. Because we had gags in our mouths it made us dribble all over. It was hilarious. The whole shoot lasted about four hours and by the end of it we were all covered in rope marks.

We made our way back to the station, staggering everywhere and giggling about the day's events. We were pretty pissed at that point and struggled to even walk in a straight line. The journey should have taken about one hour, so we should have been home by 8pm. We didn't get home until 11pm, because we got on the wrong train and ended up miles away. Good job we were so pissed that we could see the funny side.

What's your scariest moment?

The scariest moment I have ever had was when I was about 16. I went down to Essex to meet a couple of friends, who I had met on holiday. My dad drove me down halfway and my friends picked me up and we drove to their place.

I stayed there for about four days and it was really good fun. However, I was dreading going back home as I had to get the train on my own. Everything started off fine. My friends travelled to London Euston with me and put me on the train and off I went to Milton Keynes. Well, I thought I was on the train to Milton Keynes, until the train reached its destination and stopped.

There was nobody in my carriage apart from a strange man who had been staring at me all the way to wherever I was. I phoned my friend in a panic and told him that he had put me on the wrong train. I then rang my parents to tell them what had happened, but before they could offer any suggestions my battery went dead. So there I was stuck on a train in the middle of nowhere with a strange man staring at me.

I just sat in the carriage, not knowing what to do for the best. I was really scared. After about 30 minutes the train started to move back in the direction that it had come from, so I started to feel relieved. After about one hour I was back where I had started.

When I got back to Euston, I got off the train and ran as fast as I could to see if I could find someone to help me get on the right train.

KACIE LOU

Luckily I found a really nice man, who had been looking out for me. My mum had phoned the station and explained that I had got on the wrong train and I was lost. This nice man set me on my way back home and eventually I reached Milton Keynes train station. As I stepped on to the platform I was met by my mum and dad. I was so relieved I cried. That was one adventure I will never forget.

Have you ever turned down work and why?
I have only ever turned work down that I felt was not going to get me anywhere. For example, amateurs that just want to take your pictures with a throw-away camera then stick them up on their wall.

Do you have a sexual fantasy?
My sexual fantasy at the moment is to be in a top nightclub in London, surrounded by hot women. All these hot women are attracted to me and flirt with me. I invite them all back to my plush hotel, where I am staying with my boyfriend. When the girls and me get back to the hotel room, my boyfriend gets the video camera out and films me having sex with all the women. I would find this such a turn-on.

TELL ME A SECRET

What's your most memorable sexual encounter?

I do have a very memorable sexual encounter – it's an encounter that has been a big secret between the two of us – until now!

I had a shoot with Jens Wikholm (Popstar), in London. It was the first time I had met Jens, but instantly thought he was gorgeous. He had long blond hair and looked kinda scruffy, but in a sexy way. He was such a nice person too and he made me feel very horny. I think this helped, because the result of the pictures was great.

When I got home I emailed him straight away to ask what he thought about me as a model and how he felt about the images etc. He was full of positive compliments. I emailed him back and was a bit flirtatious with my response. I got the shock of my life when he reciprocated the flirting. He gave me his number and we texted each other for the next few weeks.

The result of the flirtatious texting was that I was going to stay with him at his flat in London. That day arrived and I was feeling very nervous and excited. I had a shoot in London that day and had arranged to meet him afterwards. It was on my mind all day about staying with Jens. By the end of my shoot I had worked myself up into a right state. I was worried that it would cause trouble if anyone found out that he was sleeping with one of the models, so I decided not to go.

I got back to Milton Keynes and went home, all the time questioning whether or not I should have gone to his flat. I went straight up to my room, weighing up all the pros and cons of what might happen. It must have been one-and-a-half hours later when I made the decision to head back to London.

As the taxi pulled up outside his flat, my heart was racing so hard I could feel it in my throat and thought I might die of a heart attack. He came outside and paid for the cab.

At first, I was really nervous. I think he could tell because, as soon as we stepped through the door, he opened the bottle of wine. We stood in his kitchen for a while and chatted. I felt drunk even after just one glass. I suppose it was all the excitement. Then he leaned over and started to kiss me. It felt good. I could feel myself getting turned on already, even just kissing him. He lifted me on to the kitchen worktop. I could feel how turned on he was getting.

I didn't want to rush anything until I was sure I wanted to do this, so I stopped it going any further. We went into the living room and watched a couple of DVDs. It was nearly midnight before we started to get close again. I was ready for him. I knew it was exactly what I wanted. He reached for my hand and led me to his bedroom. There was wine, romantic music and grapes on the bed, baby oil and silk sheets. At this point I was unbelievably turned on and just melted in his arms. The night was amazing. It was like something out of a romantic novel and he treated me like a queen. I will never forget it.

What do you think about group sex? Have you tried it?
I quite like the idea of group sex as long as it was all women. I have only ever had a couple of threesomes, but they weren't great. I think it was mainly because we were drunk and I was quite close to the people I was doing it with. I will give anything a try once though.

What advice would you give to someone who wanted to get into this business?
To get into the glamour industry or any modelling industry you have to be a strong person and always ready to give it your all. You cannot just give 99% effort, it has to be 110% and no less, otherwise you will find yourself getting nowhere. I have learned that you really have to want this or you won't make it work. It has to be something that you feel in your heart.

KACIE LOU

Which bloke do you fancy the most?
Vin Diesel.

Tell me a secret ... Guilt is an awful secret to live with. It never disappears from your mind. It torments you, but you keep it covered up and let it eat away at you. You can feel guilty about all kinds of things, from having a secret affair to eating that cream cake you know you shouldn't have had, because it doesn't fit in with your new healthy lifestyle. My guilt had much more traumatic consequences than a relationship break-up or gaining a few extra pounds.

Even just talking about it now I feel a lot of pain, but I'm going to tell it from the heart. I want people to know how serious drink, drugs and driving are.

It was August 2004. I was in Milton Keynes at a studio working with my best friend, Natz, who was also a model at the time. We were having so much fun mucking around and drinking while we were making video footage for our websites.

By the time we had finished the shoot we were both a bit merry. I was in the mood for having more fun, so asked Natz if she fancied going out. She didn't know whether to come out, so I said that I would go home and wait for her call. Two hours later Natz called and said that she had decided that she would come out after all.

TELL ME A SECRET

I was out for a few hours with some other friends before Natz met up with us at 11pm. We were in a gay bar called Pink Punters and in full spirits. Natz had just started her new office job and was telling us all about it. She was really loving it.

After about an hour of drinking in the bar, we decided to leave and go clubbing in central Milton Keynes, which was about a 10-minute drive from where we were. Her friends drove us, as they hadn't been drinking. We did a bit of a crawl on our way into the centre, stopping at a few pubs and clubs.

We ended up at Oceana, which is the biggest club in Milton Keynes. We had a really good time. Natz knew tons of people in Milton Keynes and I kept losing her as she went off to talk to everyone. It was disappointing when we had to leave at 3am, after the lights came on in the club.

Natz had introduced me to a few of her other friends earlier in the night and they said that they were going back to one of their houses to carry on the party. She didn't want to go on her own, so she asked if I would come.

At first I agreed, but when we got outside I decided that I didn't want to go, so I told Natz that I would just go and get a taxi. I started to head for the taxi rank, when a few of her friends came after me and said that they would drop me home. I agreed to the lift, as I didn't want my friend to be on her own.

I got into the back of the car – it was a tight squeeze as there were a few of us. The person who was driving was scaring me. He was driving really fast. We were all shouting for him to slow down, but he didn't. We finally got to my stop and I was relieved to get out. I tried to persuade Natz to come with me, but she didn't want to. The car sped off so fast I thought they were going to hit something.

It wasn't until the following day that I heard the news from a friend, who thought I had already heard. Ten minutes after I was dropped off, there had been a terrible accident. Two people had lost their lives – one of them was my best friend Natz.

I had lost her forever, all because of drink driving. I will never forgive myself that night. I was the one who persuaded her to come out that night, even though she didn't want to. If only I had insisted more that she got out of that car and stay with me, instead of letting her go off with a drink driver who was obviously not in control of the car. That 'if only' would have made sure she would still be here with us now. Natz had just turned 18 and her modelling career was just taking off. She had everything to live for. She will be missed forever.

'NATZ'
(NATALIE BLACKBURN)
3 JULY 1986 – 21 AUGUST 2004

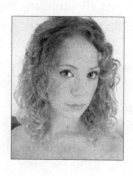

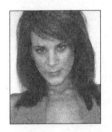

EMMA LOUISE

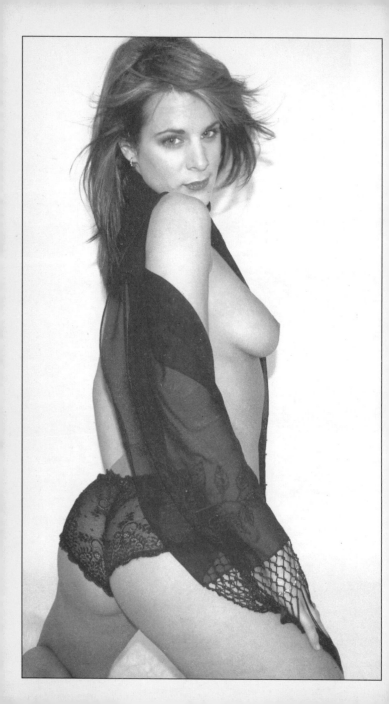

EMMA LOUISE

Name: Emma
Model/Dance Name: Emma Louise
Star Sign: Leo
Age: 23
Vital Stats: 34C-24-34
Lives: Stoke-on-Trent
Fave Food: Italian
Fave Drink: Chablis, Archers and lemonade

Where do you work?

I work at various places – the New York Table Dance at Kultfabrik is a great club, if in a strange location. Kultfabrik is now a complex of clubs, restaurants and bars, in what used to be an industrial estate. It's worth a visit, and you just follow the signs from Munich's Ostbahnhof. The club isn't like any other club that I have worked at. The entertainment is based very much around a large stage, with lots of regular shows from the girls – and boys as well as 'house parties', where everybody gets up to dance, including the customers. A bizarre experience but definitely worth a visit.

Other countries I have worked in are Norway, Spain (Mallorca) and Paris – the String Show bar in Oslo, Heaven in Magaluff, and, my favourite, Stringfellows in Paris. I have also worked in Stringfellows, London, but (please don't be offended, Peter) Paris is a totally different concept. I don't think it has anything to do with the girls, the venue, the management or the customers, but being in Paris or being Parisian seems to change the mood of the night – or something like that – it's difficult to describe. Julian who operates the Paris club once said, 'In Paris there is a club you can visit and meet your girlfriend, another where you can meet her mother, but in Stringfellows – you can meet your wife.' Paris is such a great city and we visit a few times a year just to do a bit of shopping on the Champs Elysees or, a little less expensive, sit and waste time outside a street café watching the world go by.

There are lots of other countries I want to visit – Ireland, Portugal, I must see New York and some other parts of Germany. I will write a big list and keep ticking them off till my boobs sag.

How did you get into modelling?
I was 18 when I first went to a lap-dancing club. We were in London with a group of friends for a trade show. After the show we had a night out and were on the guest list at Stringfellows. I had always been interested to see what it was like and got a great introduction to it.

My fella and his mates kept buying dances for me – perverts. I wouldn't tell them I really enjoyed it and only 'forgave' them because they were filling me with D.P. (That's the Champagne not double penetration.) After that I was hooked. A few months later we were in Dublin and I visited a really shady club in the city to do a bit more 'research'. It was dirty, tatty and full of dubious-looking people. I didn't fancy any of the girls – remind me never to work there!

Shortly after, we found out that a friend of a friend was opening their own club in Stoke-on-Trent and, as I liked the thought of the job, I went along for a look. The following week I went to have a chat with the house mum and ended up nearly naked on the stage in a horrible old pair of big knickers – dancing for her. I hated it because I wasn't expecting to go and dance, I only went to talk to her about it. I must have done OK because, three days later, I was working my first shift.

I would love to be able to tell you how I felt on my first night but having put two bottles of wine inside me before I went on ... I was a bit numb, made £70 and puked up in the car on the way home.

What's the biggest fee/tip you have ever earned?

The best was 1,900 Euro. It took until 7am to get it. It was the hardest night I have ever done but not really because of work. I had just flown out to Paris on the Monday morning. I worked Monday night straight off the plane and Tuesday night, then, straight after work in the early hours of Wednesday morning, had to get the Eurostar back to England for a family funeral at 10am. After the gathering back at the house, I had to get back on the Eurostar to Paris. Go directly to work, do not pass go, do not collect £200 and then – we got a big spender in. I hadn't slept for days and I don't think I was the best company – or looking too hot! But he kept digging into his wallet. Nice bloke!

What famous people have you danced for?

I tend to be really bad at recognising people in the flesh. Last night it took me five minutes to realise

EMMA LOUISE

I was with Darius in a club. I do remember Wes Brown, but couldn't tell you which team he played for. Phil 'The Power' Taylor – the world's most successful darts champion – keeps coming back for more. I am not really impressed by 'celebrity'. To me they are either doing a job or on a night off – so I give them a break when they are not working. It's a bit like my job. OK, so I will undress for anyone at work, but I close the curtain on the changing room when I'm trying on clothes in a shop. Most of the celebs I meet are really nice people, I would always ask before I sold a story – we all like publicity!

I could not confirm or deny that I danced for Robbie's dad last week, or that I was his only dancer that night. I believe he is a really nice guy too.

What other work have you done?
My full-time job is lap dancing. I do a few modelling jobs but not enough to feed and clothe myself. A lot of the stuff I do is for my website www.dancing.me.uk; it's good experience for me and is great for an online CV and portfolio. When I speak to a club about working for them I just direct them to the site and most say yes straight away.

I have just finished doing a calendar shoot for

my main club – ST1, along with a few of the other regular girls. They put me and my friend Becky as the cover shot – it's a really nice photo – as well as having a page inside, so I'm quite flattered. I'm Miss August, my birthday month. Buy one at www.st1-lapdancing.com.

Over the last two weeks I have done a shoot in the back of a limo with four girls for a newspaper advert and some naughtier stuff for a club website.

I spent a day at the printers last week with three other girls – smearing ink over each other's tits for some corporate Christmas cards. We did some 'tit prints' on paper as well to auction off for charity.

I am about to launch my own mobile phone web portal. The last few weeks have been taken up doing shoots for that, so there is exclusive material online for people to view. So far there are over 300 new shots of strips and pole dances as well as some fetish stuff. We are doing the girl/girl sets next so that should be a bit more fun.

I came back from a studio two weeks ago having been shackled to a cross on a dungeon wall – wearing a chain mail bikini. It was freezing in there and we had to warm the 'clothes' over a gas fire before I could put them on. The results were really good though and you can see the strange and uncomfortable clothes at www.geocities.com/alternativecostumedesign. I was in *Loaded* magazine for the first (and hopefully not the last) time in December 04, but I am not really keen on the pictures. They were taken in a rush for a deadline – as one of the country's sexiest showgirls.

What other work have you done?
When I first left school I was a chambermaid for a while in a small Scottish Bed & Breakfast Hotel – I didn't have to wear the kinky uniform as much for that as I do for my current job!

It was in my hometown, the pay was crap and I was never going to see the world doing that. I really enjoyed it though. I left Dumfries and moved to live with my auntie in Manchester. All my family lived round there; it was only really my dad and Co. who moved to Scotland. I got a job in a pickle factory – it was shite and I didn't stay long. My next job was as a chef in a busy bar just off Deansgate in Manchester. I enjoyed that – I did an NVQ and moved on to the bar too. It was a favourite haunt of lots of Manchester City players as well as lots of TV celebs – as it was round the corner from Granada Studios.

After an enjoyable time there I sadly had to leave. I had moved in with my boyfriend in South

Cheshire and the travelling was taking up half my life and all my money. I got a job at a restaurant close to my new home but then disaster struck. (I can't talk too much about this because there is still a court case pending.) To cut a long story very short – I now have two large scars on my arm. One following a serious burn and the other following the skin graft I needed. I know it affects some jobs I do but luckily most photography is digital so my scars can be easily removed with a little computer technology. I wear camouflage make-up for my dance work.

I was unemployed while I healed, got over some of the mental stress and haven't had a 'proper' job since, although I did spend nine months on a college course studying interior design.

Do you have any famous friends?

Yes, but I will leave them alone. I wouldn't want to compromise a relationship with anyone. Their private life should be their own and it is up to them to choose to disclose if they spent the evening with a 'stripper' (although some of them are glamour models anyway). It could be real tabloid fodder for those who aren't already undressing in the papers.

I love my job and I guess in this line of work you constantly get the opportunity to dish out a bit of celeb scandal. But I do the job because I genuinely love it. It is a really good feeling to entertain a crowd even if it is just standing there with my tits out as a PR stunt at an event. It is a bit of a shock to start with – when hundreds of flashguns start going off. You never know which way to look and so many people call your name. It can be blinding and deafening but very flattering once you get into it. With mobile phone cameras now there are 100 times more photographers at an event so the crowds get very big. It's a bit like being stalked by the paparazzi – exciting, but not all the time please.

I love to work on the pole in a club; people say I am really good but I just say 'average' and try my hardest. You can get a bit lazy sometimes. I like it when the rules in a club are really strict about stage shows and you have to go on three or four times a night.

Only one thing I love more than my work is SEX – I love sex so at least I guess I'm normal. You can't beat spending afternoons in the Jacuzzi at home – with a packet of fags and a bottle of Champagne, oh. and Dan, my fella, can come too if he wants. We haven't really 'tried it out' properly yet, because up until recently the neighbours could see into the back garden. Since then we have built a new fence so watch this space for some hot-tub action!

What does your family think of the work you do?
I was a bit worried about telling them at first. My mum thought it was great from the very beginning. She got really excited when I first told her and she is really proud of me – and jealous. She wants to learn to pole dance but sadly she isn't a size 8!

My dad was a bit worried to start with, about security and safety – dad stuff. I can tell he is proud. He was a bit shocked when my picture started appearing in newspapers and magazines. I can see him now at work with his mates – 'Hey Fred, isn't that …?' But he soon got over that when he realised it was OK. Wait till he reads this! My boyfriend does nothing but help and support me. He thinks it's really funny that men are so sad to give away money for nothing – but then he does have the lovely me at home. He is also really proud and says it has reinvented me – I think that's a good thing. He wishes he had tits – we could be going to Thailand for a different reason!

I enjoy going back home to visit the family in Scotland. It doesn't happen very often because of pressure of work, but, when we do, we do the family thing and then go out 'roon the toon' with the old gang. We went just last week and I discovered they had installed a pole in the local nightclub for a competition. We know the DJ there and, as I was really pissed, I couldn't resist talking him into letting me go on for a couple of tunes. I know I am a show-off but it was great to do it for a 'home crowd'.

What's your funniest moment?
I think funny is when a bloke gives you £60 for a pair of £1.99 knickers – how sick is that?

I get some funny email too. This came from Poland:

My name is *******. I am fond of stripteas. I know that this seems banal, trite, rude etc, etc. Every man, of course if he is a true guy likes stripeas and strippers. This is natura. But my interests are more widler. I love all strippers from the time when I saw stripteas my first time. It was many years ago, but my love is still very strong. I must explain you – why so do I like strippers very much. Why do I respect and admire strippers so much? In my opinion strippers are not only a symbol of sex and love, but also they are a symbol of power and victories as well. I know that this seems oddly, but look onto this problem from different side. Strippers are unusuual artists. They be able to do something great, helping oneself one's body only. They are whole naked, around them excited guys are. They are so helpless, but they are able to take controls above them. This is unusual, fascinating. This something is in kind of training of wild animals. This is not an amorous trifle, this stimultion of furious bull is. A stripper can not only to master such situation but also she is able to paralyse male mind as well. Every man are able to pay last money to her – for what – for dreams only. The single defencelles and small girl can take possession crowd of guys. This is this just magic power and it fascinates this me just. Into what way a small, gentle and naked women be able to take control above great dangerous guys. This art is unusual for me. This is a true art. I have a great dream. I want to make email conversation whit true stripper. I am looking for frank and plain girl, who likes to tell about her jobs, who likes to write letters. I want to ask many things about. I need the help. Do you want to help me?

Help him? He needs more than me to help him! You could probably add that to the scary moment section too!

Another memorable hilarious time was at God's Kitchen Global Gathering. The lap-dance venue was in a marquee in the field. It didn't get off to a good start when they realised they had lost the pole! So not many stage shows went on that night, but it did have the potential to be a really good gig and we tried our best. 35,000 captive customers to hand and an opportunity to work from 11pm 'til 6am, but it didn't really work out properly. As well as losing the pole they didn't think about the flooring very much. Can you imagine trying to walk wearing 6-inch stilettos on GRASS! Well, I did try at the beginning – for the first three minutes – but it was ridiculous. We were pissing ourselves laughing and gave up before anyone broke their ankle. I spent the rest of the evening attempting to look graceful; not a hair out of place, beautiful make-up, a long black and flowing see-through dress and a shitty pair of trainers that I had worn to drive to the gig. It was a laugh from start to finish but I made it through the whole night and made a few quid too.

What's your scariest moment?
None really, apart from the occasional email from

someone who is obviously sick in the head. Oh yeah and I can see another scary moment in the near future – when my dad reads this book!

Have you ever turned down work and why?

I turn down work all the time. A lot of requests come through from my website – wanting to take pictures of me, which is great for portfolio building but so many people ask. I would only consider this for photographers that I know personally. Many people want models for porn. This usually means come round, get naked and get shagged. I don't have a market for this stuff, but it will be great to do. I am afraid that is not for me. I do a little girl/girl action, which is fine as a show in a club, but not just shagging in a hotel room for some pervert (boyfriend excluded).

I have a request section for a bit of fun on my website. Some suggestions are really strange – a food fight – dressing as a baby – piss and poo are unprintable and this came through this morning:

> If you could poss, with nothin on, stand like a star pointing with a dirty look holding one of your breasts, not covering just on the bottom, but i wanna see u completely nude cause you are very beautiful i would like you

to personally send me these pictures i would like that very much.

I could fill the whole page with weird stuff but some ideas are OK and it is quite good to make you more versatile and keeps it fresh.

I often get asked to do escort jobs. These requests are usually from rich businessmen wanting to spend the weekend with me – 'I can afford the fees' – but I just wouldn't want to take the risk. I think that is stupid, especially when they discover they aren't going to get a shag, who knows how they would react!

I get lots of requests to go to Italy to work and spend some quality time with some male admirers. I get more mail from Italy than any other country. I don't know why.

Do you have a sexual fantasy?

If we ever visited Thailand, most of it would be for the culture, the buildings, the climate and the food. But the thought of being 'looked after' by half a dozen expert young ladies must feel great and be worth a few dollars. My bloke obviously is fully in favour of this – we have discussed it, so I can see it becoming a reality sooner, rather than later.

My ladies in waiting could bathe me, massage

me, kiss me all over and make love to me without wanting to jump in and shag straight away like a man would! Wonder where our next holiday will be ...?

What's your most memorable sexual encounter?
Have you ever had sex in a tent? It's great.

Here's one I remember oh so well. We were on holiday, doing a tour of Italy earlier last year and stayed for a couple of nights in San Marino – one of the nicest places I have ever visited (and not part of Italy). I don't know if I was especially horny because we were staying in a hotel with the Italian football teams AC Milan and Juventus (I have just thought of a new fantasy). The restaurant was full of footballers and, as it was out of the tourist season, there weren't many other guests. I was the only 'totty' in the building with 40 footballers, who didn't take their eyes off me all night. Dan and I had a nice meal, a couple of bottles of wine and then went up to bed. The footie teams were looking at my ass as we walked out of the restaurant. The atmosphere and the setting were great and there was no rush. Dan took a few photos of me because he has some kind of fetish. It was one of the few times that it was romantic and filthy at the same time. It lasted for hours. I lost count of how many times I came. I was sore in the morning but in all the right places.

What do you think about group sex? Have you tried it?
I think it's a good thing if you do it sensibly – you should see my secrets at the end!

In the right situation, happening naturally, there is no harm in it and I have never regretted it. Girls are great, a lot more sensual and erotic than blokes. I have never wanted to have it with lots of men. My bloke keeps offering to return the 'favour' but I'm not really interested. I would do it if he really wanted us to, but straight blokes don't really like to 'cross swords' too much do they and, anyway, one lot of goo is messy enough isn't it!

What advice would you give to someone who wanted to get into this business?
Do it. Do it professionally and make the most of it. Look after your money – you will only have a great body until … Never give too much of the real you away. It's good to be honest, but there must be something extra special left at home. Do I sound really mature and boring now? It is only acting with a bit of ballet thrown in. I would definitely let my daughter do it. It is as respectable and decent as YOU make it.

TELL ME A SECRET

Which bloke do you fancy the most?
Mel Gibson

Tell me a secret ... I didn't think I was a person to keep many secrets, as I prefer to be honest about things, but now you come to mention it there are a few. I hope I don't get myself, or anyone else, into trouble over this. I need some more wine first!

I am sure I am not the only girl to do this but ... when a customer is being a tosser, trying to touch you, pulling silly faces while you are dancing and licking their lips in what they *think* is a really seductive way (it is not), they really piss me off. I carry on with my dance and make sure they get a really nice view of my arse while I pull my thong down – then I fart! It just makes everything feel so much better. Dickheads beware, don't pull silly faces, you just look a twat. (I'll probably get some sick face-farting fetishists queuing for dances now I've told you that.)

There's more ... Remember I said earlier about my fantasy with my gang of Thai girls? Well, one night after a group of us had been for a night out, we got really drunk; a friend of mine and her girlfriend couldn't get a taxi home and were stuck without a lift. Dan and I offered them a bed at our house, which they accepted and we all went back for some more to drink. It wasn't long before the conversation turned to sex – lesbians and men are just the same like that – and one thing led to another. I had only ever slept with one girl before, so to end up with the three of us girls rolling round on the floor was amazing – with Dan on the side taking pictures! He was feeling a bit left out so it wasn't long before he joined the three of us. Everybody shagged ME and it was great. I said earlier that I didn't regret that kind of thing and I wouldn't normally make a habit of it but ... two weeks later we did it all again and I liked it even more because it was pre-arranged and not so much of a surprise. That bit isn't the confession. I said earlier that I loved sex and I told you that I'm not a lesbian, well this is where I have to apologise to Dan.

Dan works away from home a few nights a week and, although I would never swap him for my girlfriends, he doesn't know, until he reads this, about all the other times I have got together with my girlfriends since then and had some proper – man-free – nights in. Thanks, girls – sorry, Dan.

We had another visitor staying at our house one night, a man, but a very strange man. Do you remember the weirdo who gatecrashed Prince William's 21st Birthday Party? Shortly before the royal incident, we were all working together in a nightclub close to my home. After the gig, we went to the opening night of a friend's club for a few too many drinks. The weird one came too – he had come up on the train and couldn't get back to London 'til the morning. The strangest man in the world was staying in our house and we were scared. He slept in the spare room but we lay awake most of the night worried about what he would do. The only thing he ate while he was with us was peanut butter. He made us stop at a garage so he could stock up. Now here's the thing, a reporter from the *Sunday Sport* asked me for a few comments about this guy and what I actually said to the reporter was (you have to cash in on these things, don't you?), 'We could have woken up to find he had stolen everything or done a shit in the sink.' The reporter must have misheard me and the headline ended up 'WILLS' INTRUDER SHAT IN OUR BATH'. But, at the end of the day, I made a few quid, the nutcase got some more publicity – and the *Sunday Sport* printed some more pictures of my tits.

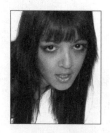

FILIZ RUSSO

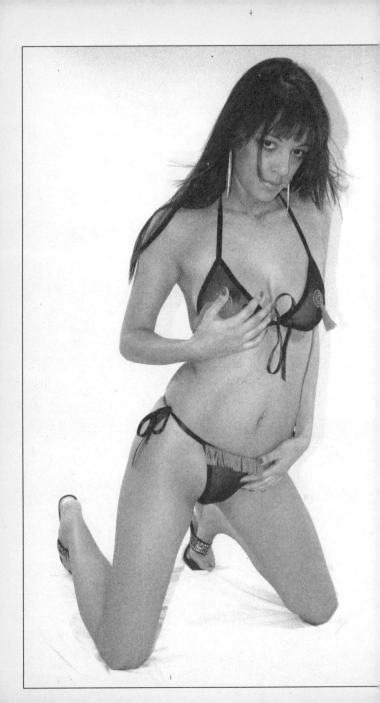

FILIZ RUSSO

Name: Filiz Russo
Model/Dance Name: Filiz Russo
Star Sign: Aries
Age: 22
Vital Stats: 32C-28-30
Lives: London
Fave Food: Turkish
Fave Drink: Cold Bud

Where do you work?

I mainly work in London but I will travel worldwide if the work's there. Actually I love travelling and it's nice to have a break from 'mad' London sometimes, but you have to be really careful. There are so many dodgy people that try things on with you, but there's nothing like a good kick in the nuts to sort them out.

TELL ME A SECRET

How did you get into modelling?

I got into modelling when I was 16. I used to do shoots behind my mum's back – they were only fashion shoots, no boob shots or anything. I always loved being in front of the camera. I was an A* drama student at school at the time, when I randomly got entered in a modelling competition when I was 18. This was when I told my mum and she just said, 'Go for it.'

I was really shocked by my mum's reaction, because my mum is very strict and so is my family. I never really took modelling seriously until I was 20. I hated doing fashion shoots, but I loved showing my body off. I felt more sexy than pretty, so I broke it to my mum gently that I wanted to do topless work. Well perhaps not that gently – I showed her a topless picture of me in the paper – oooooops!

I have had so much more confidence since I have been doing topless work. As well as a lot of pointless relationships on the way, but I feel if you have got it, flaunt it, why not? God, I'm such an exhibitionist! Ha ha!

What's the biggest fee/tip you have ever earned?

£1,000 just for an amateur shoot. Great, hey? And I only had to get my tits out.

FILIZ RUSSO

What highstreet publications have you been in?
I have been in lots of middle-shelf magazines such as *Front*, *Ice*, the *Sport*, as well as Lovers' Guide calendars, postcards, Television X, and Hollywood TV.

What other work have you done?
Well, I started modelling young but I have had loads of other jobs in between; I was a dental nurse for two years; I worked in retail and have always worked behind the bar. The first one I worked in was a gay bar. That was an experience. I loved it. It was great fun. I sometimes thought I loved bar work more than modelling, but then, when I got in front of the camera, I felt complete again.

I am currently a Tequila girl two nights a week. I started being a Tequila girl about a year ago and I love it. Basically the job involves me having to wear a sexy little outfit and selling shots of tequila slammers, which you carry around on a bullet belt. You have the glasses in one pocket, Tequila Gold in a pocket, as well as the bottle of lime and tabasco sauce. It's a strong shot and my job is to get everyone as drunk as possible and make lots of money.

You get to meet all sorts of characters. I work all over London, in all the nightclubs and bars. I obviously have a few favourites and I usually end up dancing the night away – oooops! Hope my boss doesn't read this! Ha ha.

In most of the clubs you are the main attraction, so it's great. People want to buy shots off you just so you stand there and chat and some of them recognise you from magazines or TV. It's great when you get a group of lads because they're always up for it, especially if you flirt a bit with them. I wait till they're all really drunk and then I attack, ha ha. I pour the shots, get them all to slam, blow the whistle and they're off. Before you know it they are up for another shot.

The funniest moment I have had doing tequila work was when I was working at a bar in east London. A group of guys bought a round of shots and after they had done their first round, they were all fine and then they thought that they would be brave and buy a second round straight after. Well, one of the guys who did the second shot ended up throwing his guts up on the table in his friends' drinks, in front of the whole bar. It was really horrible to watch. I made him clean the lot up. Unfortunately, I didn't sell much after that – not sure why!

Do you have any famous friends?
I have one celebrity friend, which is Jo Guest. I

met her at a party and did a punk aid video with her. We have also appeared together in the paper. She is so lovely. I think we get on so well 'cause she is a lot like me, a bit of a ladette.

What does your family think of the work you do?
Well, the only family I have is my mum, sister and little brother; the rest are all losers. They hate what I do and I hate what they do to my mum. My mum always sticks up for me. She was brought up in a strict Muslim family, you know, the ones where the daughters had to bring up four brothers and three sisters, while her dad just shouted out orders and beat her when he felt like it.

My uncles think they can do the same to me. They took everything from us and left us with nothing. Now they have nothing and we are all really happy. As they say, what goes around comes around.

What's your funniest moment?
I was with an ex-boyfriend and we were in the car outside my house one night and we were getting all horny. So we decided to drive to One Tree Hill for a bit of car sex. Everyone in Essex goes there to shag.

We were on the car bonnet, and he was on top. The next thing I know is that there were really bright car lights in front of me. I quickly pulled my knickers up and then noticed it was the police. We thought we might be in trouble or get done for indecent behaviour or something. But they wound down the window, had a good butchers and let us carry on. It turned me on being watched by a couple of men in uniform, so we did carry on. We even had some guy walk past with his dog and we didn't stop. I think we kept a few people happy that night.

What's your scariest moment?

When I went to a fortune teller who told me my that my dad was there. That was some really freaky shit and scared the hell out of me.

It was all a bit much; she said a lot of things that were true and it scared me a lot. She had mentioned a few things about my dad, who had passed away, so I was very worried about talking about him. Then she said to me, 'If I told you your dad was here would you believe me?' and I said 'No'. The next thing she told me was something that happened with my mum a week before. It was just a random conversation, that's all and I said, 'Wow, how did you know that?' and she said, 'The only reason I know that is because your dad is standing here telling me.' I was so shocked I did not know what to say to that. I do believe her and I do believe that fortune tellers are gifted people, but there are some people that take it for granted or just talk bullshit. My mum is a spiritual person and she always gives me advice or guides me. She is really good at predicting things and I never used to believe in anything like that, but I do now.

Have you ever turned down work and why?
I have learned that you should always trust your gut feeling in this industry. There was one time when I didn't and it turned sour, so if people contact me on the net and ask me to shoot I always make sure they hire a studio first, so I feel safe. There have been a few times I have said no and other models have told me they had done it and ended up having a very bad shoot and were put in a very scary situation.

I do not understand why girls would just go and shoot with anyone, as there are so many nutters about. I think that every girl in the industry has had a bad experience. I think I'm very lucky not to have experienced anything too scary.

Do you have a sexual fantasy?
My fantasy sounds so dirty, but I would love to hitch hike and have a really sexy lorry driver stop to give me a lift. We'd end up having wild

sex in the lorry ha ha – God, that sounds filthy.

The reason why I would love to have random sex with a lorry driver is because it would be so naughty. I would have to be wearing thigh-high boots, short skirt and a little bra top. It would have to be really hot weather (not asking for much, hey?) and I would be wearing crotchless knickers.

The lorry driver would have brown hair, green eyes and be wearing one of those American-style sleeveless shirts with muscles pounding out. I would have to straddle him, with just my skirt lifted so we could have dirty sex with my crotchless knickers on. It would be really dirty sex, really sweaty and everyone could see us. Then I would get him to drop me off home for a nice cup of tea and a Yorkie, ha ha!

What's your most memorable sexual encounter?

My best sexual encounter was with my boyfriend. We were in Amsterdam for a dirty weekend for Valentines. We smoked loads of wacky backy and the hotel played constant porn for the four days we were there. It was great, we had a major shag session and it was the fourth time having sex that night and I had the best orgasm ever. It was bliss.

FILIZ RUSSO

What do you think about group sex? Have you tried it?
I know loads of girls that have done it and they love it. I think, if I was going to have a go, I would prefer two girls and a guy and the other girl would have to be really gorgeous and I would have to be very drunk.

What advice would you give to someone who wanted to get into this business?
It's a great industry to get into, providing you do it right. For instance, if I had a daughter I would let her do it, but I would make sure she had a good head on her shoulders. I would start her off young in kids agencies to get her used to it and I would give her a choice.

My advice to anyone who wants to start modelling is make sure you have a good portfolio, get a good agent and never leave the country without anyone. Trust yourself in this industry, not anyone else, and don't let anyone try and push your limits. Never do shoots in hotels or people's homes and always ask for references. You are the one at risk, remember that.

Which bloke do you fancy the most?
Kurt Cobain

TELL ME A SECRET

Tell me a secret ⋯ I'm not sure if the other girls that were involved with this event are going to be happy about me telling all, but here goes.

I had been talking to this guy on the internet for about a year. He was a well-known American photographer. His work was absolutely amazing. He had mentioned for a few weeks that he was coming to London to cast some girls for a calender shoot for an American Athlete's team. It was a big job and all the girls would get paid mega bucks. So, knowing how much of a great photographer he was, me and two other model friends, went along to the casting in London.

He did some really nice shots of us and he decided to book all three of us. We were all really pleased. We had two days to get our things ready. But one of the girls decided last minute that she wanted to go on a different flight to us a few hours earlier. Me and the other model went together later that day.

As I got on the plane, I had a really funny feeling. My mum and boyfriend had told me not to go, but I didn't listen. But, then again, when I was on the plane, I had a really strong gut feeling that something wasn't right. I tried to shake it off and a few drinks on the plane helped!

When we got there we had been booked in to a lovely hotel. However, when we checked in, we discovered that I was sharing with the model who had arrived earlier that day and my friend, who I had travelled with, was on her own. Apparently the hotel had been told specifically who was to have their own room. Funnily enough, he had taken a bit of a liking to the model he booked into her own room. She was a bit uneasy about this situation, so I offered to share with her so she felt safe.

We went to see the other girl, who was in bed at the time. She said that the photographer had come into her room and asked her if she'd ever considered escorting, or doing open-leg work. She was really shocked and told him 'no way'. She found him really creepy and his assistant, a girl, was even more creepy. He kept on telling us that his assistant fancied one of us. We were all really freaked out by this, and I was really upset that I never trusted my gut feeling. I had always done before.

The next day all three of us were feeling very nervous about the real reason why he had got us over here. If that wasn't enough evidence to be feeling scared, he also brought four massive sportsmen up to our bedroom while we were getting changed. I thought this was a bit pervy and very much out of order.

As soon as we managed to get rid of the guys

out of our room, I phoned my agent. I wanted to find out if there was any more information about this guy. I explained about what he had said to my friend and the four sportsmen he brought up to our bedroom.

We still went to the casting, but it was very obvious that he just wanted sexy girls there for these athletes that were there. While we were still at the casting my agent called back. She told us to get our things and get out of there as soon as we could. Apparently this guy was all over the news and he was alleged to have drugged models and pimped them out. He was also sending them to Arabia to get rid of them.

As soon as I put the phone down I grabbed the other two girls. We made our excuses why we needed to go back to the hotel. We quickly packed our stuff and escaped through the fire exit. Our hearts were racing, as we clambered down nine flights of stairs. We were scared. We jumped in a cab and went straight to the British Embassy. We were all too frightened to say too much as we thought that something bad might happen to us. But the Embassy helped us get back to the airport and on a flight back home.

I can't mention any names, but I hope the other girls don't go mad at me for telling this story. This has got to be the worst experience of my life. I am usually really good with my gut feeling, but this time I just ignored it. We have never told anyone this story until now, so the girls are going to hate me. But it feels great to get it off my chest.

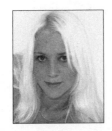

LUCKY

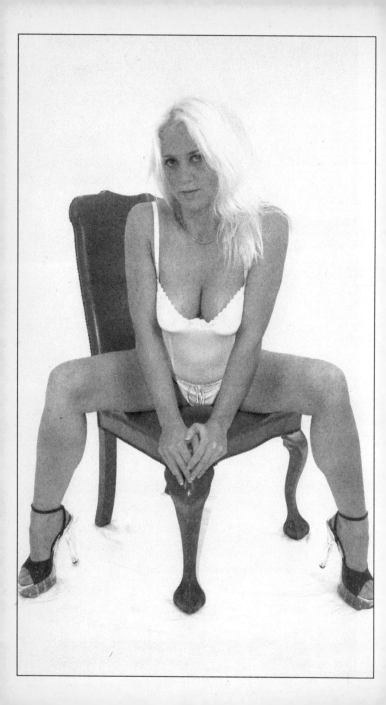

LUCKY

Name: Amanda Vrona
Model/Dance Name: Lucky
Star Sign: Pisces
Age: 26
Vital Stats: 34DD-29-34
Lives: Taunton, Somerset
Fave Food: Pasta
Fave Drink: Vodka Red Bull

Where do you work?

I am currently working at Temptations, in Union Street, Plymouth. I have been working at this club since May 2004. At the moment I work Thursday night 7pm–2am, Friday night 9pm–2am and I also do a double shift on Saturday 12.30pm–2am.

The club is really nice; it used to be a casino which they turned into a lap-dancing club. It has a huge stage with two rotating poles and floor tiles that light up. It has a VIP lounge, table dance room and loads of dance booths. All the girls in the club are great and they all get on with each other, even the management. This is probably one of the friendliest clubs that I have ever worked in.

How did you get into dancing?

I got in to this line of work through my boyfriend, Rich. He was working in London and his local pub was a strip pub. When I went to visit him he took me into the pub to see the girls and they told me I'd be fine to give it a go. They told me how much money they earned, who to ring and where to go for an audition.

I got my first 'live' audition for the Rainbow Sports Bar in Shoreditch High Street, London. I had to be there for 9pm on a Monday night. My boyfriend drove me and we were running late, which made me feel even more scared and unprepared.

The audition had been booked through an agency called Rainbow International Ltd and the bar was owned by them. Anyway, I downed a couple of drinks, did the strip and passed the audition. They basically said that I had the job and if I stopped shaking I would do fine.

When I was stripping at the club, I would walk

around the customers collecting money in a jug, then go on stage when I thought there was enough in the jug to do my strip.

The agency had loads of pubs all over London, Kent, Middlesex and Surrey, with about 200 girls rotating around the pubs. So that's how I started stripping in London.

The next stage was to become a lap dancer, which is what I do now and I have lap danced in London, Cardiff, Bournemouth, Swindon, Salisbury and now Plymouth. Lap dancing is different to stripping, as you take turns on the stage promoting yourself and then you charge the customers for private dances: £10 topless, £20 nude and the only jugs on show are your own!

Aside from the club work I have also done a topless challenge for the *Daily Sport* and have been in *Redline* magazine as a runner-up of a Beach Babe competition.

What's the biggest fee/tip you have ever earned?

My biggest night of earning was at Spearmint Rhino, Bournemouth. It was a busy Saturday night and my take-home pay, after paying commission, in one shift was £600. That was doing lap dances and VIPs all night.

TELL ME A SECRET

What famous people have you danced or modelled for?

I worked with Jordan at Spearmint Rhino in Bournemouth. She came down to do a promotions night. Jordan was taught to pole dance during the day for her shows at night. I was surprised at how nice Jordan was, and she was really down to earth. She kept saying to me that she doesn't know how we do our job, as she was really scared.

I had said that all the girls hated the slimy DJ that worked at the club, so, when she was interviewed by the DJ on stage, she was really funny and just took the piss out of him. All the girls thought it was great and cheered her on.

I gave an interview on Jordan and left a good luck message to the camera crew for her.

When I was working in Club Rouge in Salisbury last year I danced for someone who had just entered to be in *Pop Idol*. I can't remember his name and I don't know how far he made, it as I left the club to work somewhere else.

I danced for some lord's son in the same club. He was quite young, completely up himself, but well spoken. He would always boast about all his girlfriends and how many parties he would go to in London. Everyone knew who he was and the club always gave him credit to pay for his dances.

LUCKY

He used to make my skin crawl. The club was going downhill fast and it was starting to look more like a pub than a lap-dancing club. There was many interesting, rich, well-known and dodgy men I could talk about for hours that used to go in there.

More recently I have auditioned to dance in a music video for an American rap artist called Ralph Dog. He is staying in London to record his new album. I will also be featured on the cover of his album. I can't wait to work for him.

What other work have you done?
I've had loads of really shit jobs, like cleaning at the magistrates court, that was evening work – as if I didn't have a social life to fill my evenings. I worked in the restaurant for the Post House, Asda supermarket on the checkouts and as a care assistant. I've even been a security guard! I didn't really like any of these jobs but it paid the bills at the time – just.

I went to Kingsmead Community School and left with 10 GCSEs and two NVQs

Do you have any famous friends?
I have loads of friends, some real close. They all like what I do and are always interested in what I am going to do next. None is famous, but if I

could pick a famous friend it would probably be Jordan. She inspires me. I love what she does and her attitude towards life and, of course, I would love her fame and fortune. Although I would question her taste in some of the men she has hooked up with.

What does your family think of the work you do?

After I passed my audition in London I came home and met my mum in the local pub, the White Hart, to have a drink and that's when I first told her what I had just been doing. She was well excited; she was shouting it out in the pub telling everybody. She was more excited than I was. She wanted to know all about it – what I would have to do? How? How much money? Where? When? She did not mind one bit. She has bought me thigh-high boots for work, framed *Redline* magazine, when there was topless pics of me in it. She also has a picture hanging proudly up on the living-room wall of me and another dancer, Roxy, dressed up in sexy, saucy Santa outfits. When she has guests around she directs them to the picture and introduces me as the middle child, the lap dancer!

None of my family has been to watch because I always dance away from where I live. My sister, Natasha, really wants to come and see me. She is fascinated by it all, I have asked her to come and dance with me, but she is far too shy. My boyfriend has seen me dance and a few of my friends, but I always get a bit nervous when people are there I know, but I don't mind.

I suppose I couldn't ask for a more supportive family, they are all great.

What's your funniest moment?

My life is filled with funny moments. I think the funniest and most embarrassing moment was when I was doing a lap dance for a gentleman. It was at Club Rouge, in Salisbury. It was a big room with loads of sofas and UV lights. I started my dance and got up on the sides of the chair and when I looked down my tampon string was dangling around in front of the man's face. I was so embarrassed and because of the UV lights it stood out really badly. All the other girls dancing in the room saw it, even the doorman, who was across the other side of the room. Everyone started laughing. I got down and tucked it away quickly and carried on dancing as best I could still giggling to myself. I will never live that one down.

Another time when I was stripping in London I tripped over my knickers on stage and went flying. I got a round of applause, but I just laughed with everyone and carried on.

I sometimes wonder whether I'm maybe a bit accident-prone and, maybe, should have extra insurance for when I'm dancing. There was another time when I went to do a pole trick called the helicopter. The helicopter trick is where you climb up the pole cross your legs in front of you, then lean back so you're upside down with legs in air. On this occasion I didn't get the grip right and slid down the pole really fast and landed on my bum – that hurt! I had a massive bruise for days afterwards; it didn't look very nice and took me forever to cover it up each night.

What's your scariest moment?

My most scary moment was probably when I worked for the sports bar in Shoreditch High Street, London. There was no security there, so, when you leave, you're on your own. One night I was followed by a really tall, big-built black bloke. He started hassling me and wouldn't let me into my car. It was the early hours of the morning in the middle of London and no one was around and I didn't know anyone in the area. I had my one-year-old pitbull Rocky in the car. I use to bring her to work to protect me and to keep me company on the long drive home. I eventually managed to tell the bloke my dog was inside and that she was very friendly (not) and I needed to let her out for a wee. I managed to open the car door to let my dog out. She jumped out and sat in front of me growling at him. He eventually left me alone. I was so scared and shaking. I got my dog back in the car and tried to drive off, but my car was now playing up. I had to jump out of the car again to lift the bonnet and bleed the diesel to get it started. Then it stalled at the lights and I had to jump out of the car again. The bloke was still hanging around and I was so scared. I eventually drove off crying and phoned my boyfriend to comfort me. That was my first and most scary moment.

Have you ever turned down work and why?
I have never turned down work, but I turn men down every night I work – I have a boyfriend, no I will not meet you afterwards, no I am not interested in £50 at the end of the night. They just don't understand we are dancers not prostitutes.

Do you have a sexual fantasy?
My sexual fantasy would be to meet my man outside at night and make love in a public place. The thought of the wind brushing over our bodies while we make love and the thrill of maybe we will get caught, really turns me on.

TELL ME A SECRET

What's your most memorable sexual encounter?
I think my most memorable to date has got to be when me and my fella had sex on a beach in Spain in the early hours of the morning.

What do you think about group sex? Have you tried it?
My thoughts on group sex are, why not, you have to try everything once. Yes, I have tried it once.

What advice would you give to someone who wanted to get into this business?
My advice would be, go to a club first, have a look around and talk to some of the girls. Find yourself a nice outfit and a song you know you can dance to, this will help your confidence. Start practising your dance routine by yourself, before you go to any auditions. Use a cushion on your sofa and dance for that. If you have a boyfriend then try it out on him too. When you start feeling good about it, phone the club and ask for an audition.

Which bloke do you fancy the most?
I think Vin Diesel is fit! He is so sexy.

Tell me a secret ⋯ My biggest secret was an affair I had with another woman. I had not been working at Temptations very long, but got on great with all the girls. One night I had planned to stay at another dancer's house. We were having a good laugh and had far too many drinks. I had never had sex with another woman, but had thought about it. I guess that's why lap-dancing clubs are so popular, there is something very sexual about watching naked women dance and tease you.

When we got to the house we decided to put the TV on and watched *Men and Motors*. The programme was making me very horny. I don't know whether I imagined it, but our breathing seemed slower, louder and in time. I couldn't concentrate too much on the programme. I was aching with passion and looking at my friend, who looked so sexy.

After a while she started to rub my leg, moving to the inside of my thigh. I wasn't sure what to do, but I wanted her to know that I wanted something to happen. So I turned to her and started cuddling her. I was unbelievably turned on and we were soon kissing. It was very different kissing a girl. I remember thinking how soft and gentle her lips were. Our tongues gently touching, while her hands caressed my breasts. Then when she parted my legs with her hands I thought my body was going to explode. By the time she got to my thong, I was already well creamed. She pulled them to the side and rubbed my clit. I was moaning really loud at this time. She looked at me and smiled, and I could tell she wanted me to touch her.

I slowly lifted up her top. She had great tits, big, firm and erect nipples. I sucked her nipples, and I knew she liked it because she was holding my head and pushing me firmer on to them. I couldn't wait any longer: I needed her pussy. I pulled her gently back and opened her legs; she wasn't wearing any knickers. I licked the inside of her thighs slowly making my way to her pussy, sucking her hard little clit.

In no time she climbed on top of me and returned the favour. We were 69ing each other, licking each other's wet pussies. When I could feel her start to come, it made me come. It was a long pulsating joint orgasm. I was in heaven. After we had both come, we kissed each other and went to bed, in separate rooms. No more was ever said about it! What a night!!

I have thought about it a lot and wonder whether I would do it again. I guess it was too good not to repeat, but I would prefer my boyfriend to join in – even better!

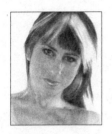

FENYA

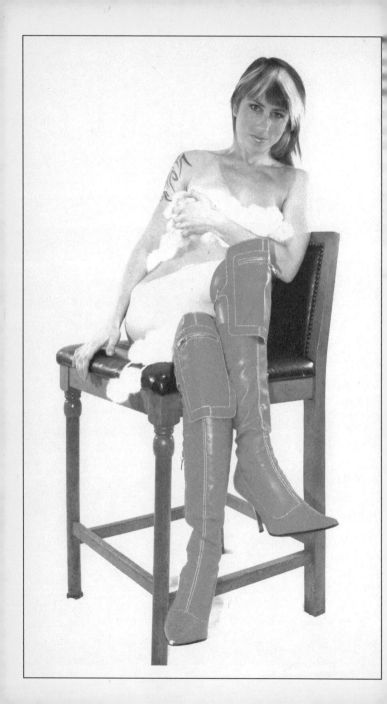

FENYA

Name: Linda Walker
Model/Dance Name: Fenya
Star Sign: Sagittarius
Age: 29
Vital Stats: 34C-26-35
Lives: Hampshire
Fave Food: Chinese
Fave Drink: Sparkling water

Where do you work?
I dance podium wherever there is work. At the moment I work locally every Saturday night. I started lap dancing but it hasn't been busy enough to earn the cash, so I'm not bothering with that until it gets busier.

I also model and do promotional work, such as *Max Power* and *Super Bikes*. I have modelled body paint – that's fun.

I travel to wherever there is work. I love bikes and have a bike licence, so working for mags such as *SuperBike* is great.

I have worked all over Ibiza for a couple of years in a row. I dance at places such as Judgement Sunday at Eden, Sundissential at Pacha, Manumission at Privilege, Club Submission at El Divinios and the water party at Esparadis. The place is amazing if you are a real party-goer. The beaches ain't great but I guess you don't go for the beaches!

How did you get into dancing and modelling?

I have a few friends that dance and model and I thought that I would like to give it a go. So they helped me by me giving numbers and agents. I called around some agents, but they are hard to find, because I have lots of tattoos. Then I started to call magazines and got some work that way. I also have dance agents and some of them put modelling work my way.

I first started my dance work because I wanted to go out to raves and couldn't afford them on my wages. I've loved dancing all my life, so, when I was 18, I phoned World Dance and got an audition with the Fetish Crew. I started to dance with them. However, they paid only now and then, but, as I was going out and having fun doing it, I didn't mind too much. Then my boyfriend at the time was telling me that he thought the agent was taking the piss. If I wasn't getting the money, then who was? So I quit and went to work for someone else that paid every time I worked. I was working closer to home four nights a week and loving it even more, because I was being paid too.

To this day, dancing makes me feel alive.

What's the biggest fee/tip you have ever earned?

I was paid £250 for one night's work, walking around as sexy Santa. It was in a pub in Essex. All we had to do was walk around a pub and chat to the people. It was fun. I was invited back this year, but I didn't make it. I was driving there and took the wrong turning and went a bit out of the way. I phoned the manager to let him know and he said not to come as we were too far away. So me and my friend had a great Christmas Eve driving around the M25! (Not!)

What highstreet publications have you been in?

I was in the *Daily Star* for going on *The Salon*, and I have modeled for the *Sunday People*, *SuperBike*, *Bizarre*. I also danced on Dance Star Awards Ibiza, at a Judge Jules Club Nite there.

TELL ME A SECRET

What other work have you done?

I'm a hairdresser and currently I'm working for Toni and Guy. I have been hairdressing 12 years now, a real golden oldie. I also worked on the Channel four programme *The Salon*.

I was a stylist cutting people's hair at the time and I applied to an ad that came to my salon, for a chance to appear on the TV programme *The Salon*. I wasn't going to apply at first because I was really nervous. But they sent an application form to my house so I filled it in and got an interview.

The next stage was a trade test, which is when you do a haircut and the judges see your work. Paul Merrit, the manager of *The Salon*, was one judge; Bev Cobralla, hairdresser of the year, was the second. Bev's hubby was the third judge. It was all very funny. I didn't think much of any of them, so it didn't put me on edge. I just got on with my cut and enjoyed it for what was it was worth. But surprise, surprise I got in!

The show itself was hard work as it wasn't about hair, but about who could be the loudest and funniest. I wanted to show off my hairdressing skills, so didn't bother playing up to the cameras, which is why I didn't have my contact renewed. Channel 4 was disappointed because I wasn't the livewire they thought I was. Oh well, it was fun at the time and I got to do a few memorable haircuts, such as Danny Dyer. Oh my God, he is lovely! And Terri Dyer, she is a star. Uri was a bit mad but lovely. The best moment was meeting 5 star and last, but not least, was doing Super Bike rider Steve's hair. I love bikes and to know he was sporting my haircut and colour was just great.

In November I am hoping to go to Australia to work for three months. Toni and Guy have branches out there, so I thought, as I'm 30 this year and you can't get a working visa over, it's now or never. I have emailed the salons and headquarters and it has all gone from there. I would also like to get some work dancing out there.

Do you have any famous friends?

I am friends with Vanessa Upon. I first worked with Vanessa in Ibiza. I was living in an apartment with her. Then a few years later, I was working for an agent and we met up again and danced together and worked at Hammersmith Trade Shows Rubberball. We have become good friends and she was bridesmaid at my wedding. I am also friends with Terry from *The Salon* and I use to do Lucy Pinder's hair.

What does your family think of the work you do?

They love it. My husband doesn't mind as long as

I'm happy. My mum loves the fact that she has something to gossip about – that her daughter does this and does that. She always said when I was a kid, that I would do Page 3. It was a bit of a joke at the time, because I never wanted boobs – God, now look at me! The bigger the better!

What's your funniest moment?
One night I was working at Ikon in Southampton, and Gary Lucy, from *Footballers Wives*, was also there doing a signing. When I finished dancing, I was hot and sweaty and he turned to me and said, 'I'd hate to think what you smell like', or something like that. So I replied, 'smell like your face', at the same time as kissing him on his cheek and rubbing my sweaty face all over his, and I ran off laughing. He was well pissed off and called me a few names. I really hate him – he is right up his own arse, so I thought it was funny, ha ha.

What's your scariest moment?
When the Pied Piper wouldn't take no for an answer, pulling me by the arm, wanting me to go upstairs. I gave him my husband's phone number to shut him up and then he left. But he got real mad when he turned up at another club I was working at a few weeks later. He was trying to

talk to me and hassling me. He was not impressed that I had given him my husband's number. When I left the club that night I was really scared. I had seen how mad he was and was shitting in case he was following me.

Have you ever turned down work and why?
Yes, I turn work down all the time if the money ain't good, then I'm not going and the clothes are staying on.

I get emails all the time from websites, wanting to shoot up my skirt first with my pants on, then being taken off.

One bloke wanted to be my slave – yeah, mate, you can come and do the ironing for my hubby and me! I always get blokes telling me I am lovely asking if they can be my boyfriend, or offers for work to do girl on girl video work. I get pissed off with the porn ones as I am not interested and would never do it. I even put a request on the website for people to stop asking.

Do you have a sexual fantasy?
My fantasy is to sleep with one of my girl friends, Vanessa Upon, but as I'm not really into girls I would love it to stay a fantasy, because my dreams are hot and it's good to have a dream.

TELL ME A SECRET

What's your most memorable sexual encounter?
All sex with my hubby is memorable. We have great sex. That's all I want to say on his matter, as I think this is something not to talk about.

What do you think about group sex? Have you tried it?
If people want to do it, well, let them, but it's not my bag as it all ends up in tears. I have some friends that tried it and it ended in tears, the couple spilt up and the other girl ended up gay. I think it's sad when you feel you have to do something like this for your man if he asks you. When he starts pressuring you to do group sex then it's time you showed him the door. Your man should love you for you, not for what you would let him do, like have his cake and eat it.

What advice would you give to someone who wanted to get into this business?
To start with you have to be a good dancer. I hate it when I have to audition someone and then have to tell them they can't dance. Ask a friend what they think before phoning an agency – harsh, I know, but how do you think I feel having to tell someone they can't dance? If you can dance, call the clubs direct and ask for the number of the agent who runs the dancers.

FENYA

For modelling do a search on net and send off pics and your CV; they will say yes or no, or call the mags and send pics to them. It's all about marketing yourself – the more you contact, the better chance you have.

Which bloke do you fancy the most?
Jean Claude Van Damme

Tell me a secret ... For years I suffered from bullying. It all started when I was nearly a teenager. It's bad enough as a teenager, having to deal with hormones etc, but to top it all I had to move schools due to family break-up.

I felt very down. I had to move to the other side of the country, leaving all my friends and familiarities. I suppose that it made me feel a bit insecure. I was only 12 and felt like I didn't have anyone.

It was upsetting dealing with the family break-up, but I tried to think of the positives and figured I would soon make friends and soon it would all be back to normal. How wrong I was – I didn't realise how nasty kids could be. Trying to make new friends in a new and alien area was the hardest thing I have ever had to do. When I finally thought I had found a friend, this so-called friend started taking the piss out of me, calling me a man-like creature, because I was a bit of tomboy and looked and acted like a boy.

Because of what I went through when I was younger and all the suffering these people caused me, it made me want to succeed as a dancer more than anything else in the world. I wanted to dance and model, just to show these assholes that people change. Even now, all these years on, I want to succeed more than ever and reach my goals and to show these nasty people that they didn't get the better of me.

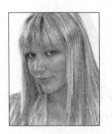

HOLLYBLUE

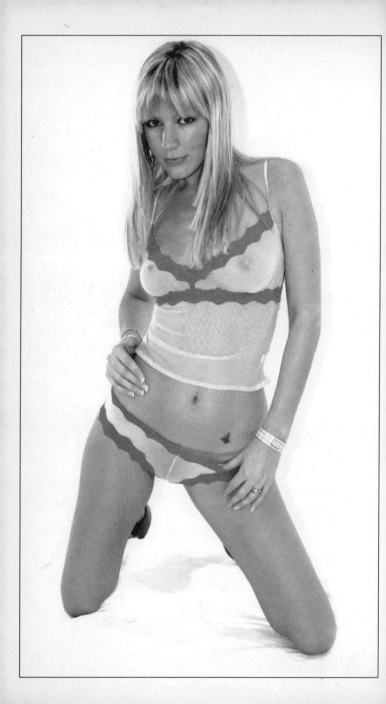

HOLLYBLUE

Name: Holly Newberry
Model/Dance Name: Hollyblue
Star Sign: Gemini
Age: 23
Vital Stats: 34B-23-33
Lives: Norfolk
Fave Food: Italian/Spanish/Roasts
Fave Drink: White wine, Caprisun

Where do you work?
I am a full-time model and do promotional work for *Max Power* Live Shows, *FHM*, *Playboy* lingerie, *Maxim*, chatline ads etc. At the moment I have only worked in the UK but am keen to travel further on assignments.

How did you get into modelling?
I used to go and model for a photographer, John

Hedgecoe, in Norfolk. He has lots of books out on photography techniques. I always wanted to do glamour, so I entered some of the photographs in a competition in the *Sunday Star* in January 2003. To my surprise I won and that got me an agent.

I wanted to model from about the age of 10. I thought it would also be good to understand the other side of the camera, so I went to college to study photography.

I used to find it frustrating waiting for my big break into modelling. I was 20 when I finally made the break, which nowadays is a lot older than most people getting into glamour.

I love modelling. I complain sometimes, but it's wicked and I wouldn't want to change my career. I love showing off my body. I love the attention, always have and always will.

What's the biggest fee/tip you have ever earned?

Not a lot – maybe when I've been modelling longer and got a name for myself it will be a lot more. I think the most so far is £400 for a one-day shoot. It was for the *News of The World*. I told them about when I was in a club and a girl came up to me and asked me to kiss her and I did. I said I'm not a lesbian and I certainly didn't do it to impress any boys around. Lots of girls do it – I was just curious, again.

HOLLYBLUE

What highstreet publications have you been in? Have you worked with any famous people?

Mainly middle-shelf mags such as *Max Power*, *Maxim*, and *FHM*, but I have also done *Playboy Lingerie*. I've also been in the *Sunday Star*, which is how I got started, and the *News Of The World*. I once did a video shoot with Darren Hayes from Savage Garden.

What other work have you done?

I studied Fashion at Norwich School of Fashion and also studied styling and photography at Greshams School in Norfolk.

I have done work experience for Nicole Farhi and Magazine(*Daily Mail*), which basically meant that I had to sit in a room sorting through clothes that the magazine had used, which they wanted to send back to the designers or PRs. I answered the phones and basically it showed me how unglamorous it all was – although it was fun at the time.

Do you have any famous friends?

I haven't any famous friends. My friends are all normal people, which suits me fine. I'm happy to go home after work to people who aren't in my industry – it's refreshing.

TELL ME A SECRET

What does your family think of the work you do?
I guess they aren't that bothered, as they are quite open people. Nudity isn't a problem in my family. Mum use to work for David Bailey so was also in the industry (mags). They don't mind so long as shoots aren't too rude or too provocative!

They weren't happy when I was topless in the *Sport*; they don't mind Playboy lingerie, *Maxim* etc. I don't blame them; I wouldn't want to see my daughter in the *Sport* topless. *FHM* wouldn't be a problem, as the pictures are tasteful, sexy not slutty.

My brother has a problem with my modelling. He is very much a businessman, selling property in Spain. His issue is he doesn't want his mates seeing me topless or nude. It embarrassed him once when he saw me getting out of a car on the cover of the *Sport*, showing my knickers. He went in a right mood and was really mad with me and demanded the photographer's number. I'm not sure what he would have done, even if I had given him the number.

What's your funniest moment?
This is probably not the funniest, but probably the most stereotypical thing I can think of.

Some other models and me were on a music video shoot for the band Phixx. We got chatting and moaning about this and that, then one of the models turned to us and said, 'Isn't it hard to just blink sometimes, such an effort.' We all looked at each other, wondering whether we had heard right. Then we fell about laughing: 'What the f*** are we like!' So f***ing pathetic – such a 'model' thing to say!

What's your scariest moment?

One scary moment was my first music video casting, which was for a Darren Hayes video, the guy from Savage Garden. I'm not a trained dancer, so, when I was asked to dance to a track in front of five people, I was really shitting myself – it was quite daunting. I also didn't realise how long I had to dance for and what was worse is they told me to dance a bit crazy, overly sexy etc. It was hard to be sexy when the tune was so poppy.

Now when I go for video castings I make sure that I can dance with a mate or any other girl who is at the casting.

Have you ever turned down work and why?

I've turned down Page 3 *Sport*, as it's so tacky – the pictures are vile. The only other work I've turned down is shoots where boys/men are in shot with me in a sexual way, as my boyfriend would get jealous and he has asked me if I wouldn't do it. So I won't.

I don't do storyboards for papers either, cos they always involve men. I wouldn't mind posing with men – really it's just work. But I don't want to upset my bloke.

Do you have a sexual fantasy?

God, I don't really have one fantasy that I go back to like I'm sure many people do. I used to constantly fantasise about meeting Brad Pitt when he was in *Legends of the Fall*, looking like a cowboy, Mmm. I just used to pretend I was his love interest in the film. Well, I was only 13 at the time, ha ha.

If I haven't seen my bloke for ages I just fantasise about everything we are going to do when I see him. It usually involves me being in a shower and being lifted up.

What's your most memorable sexual encounter?

When I started going out with someone six years ago we lived miles away from each other, so we communicated a lot by telephone. That also included a large part of our sexual relationship. We would have phone-sex all night. He would start at my mouth and fully undress me, then work his way down my body. He took ages, telling me each inch of the way what he was doing to my body. It was great!

What do you think about group sex? Have you tried it?

I haven't ever tried group sex. I think it is OK if everyone is up for it. If not, I reckon it can be awkward, but, if they are all up for it, I bet it's fantastic – more hands to pleasure you etc!

What advice would you give to someone who wanted to get into this business?

Prepare to wait for your money. Make sure you are able to support yourself in other ways until you have regular cash coming in. Keep away from any jobs that you have doubts over, as you will regret it. Everyone I know who does the *Sport* seems to really regret it, including me.

Which bloke do you fancy the most?

Brad Pitt was one of my favourites, now Johnny Depp is more to my taste – he is very cool and sexy. And my bloke of course.

Tell me a secret ··· I suppose my biggest secret that I have never told anyone was a bit of a lesbian video-filming experience I had with two other girls.

TELL ME A SECRET

I was out around London having a few drinks. I bumped into a couple of girls that I hadn't seen for a while – let's call them Sarah and Amanda.

I hadn't intended having a heavy night, but it was great seeing them both again. They were going to a model party and invited me to go along. The Champagne was flowing and we were getting pretty drunk.

When the party was over, we decided that we should go back to Amanda's place and drink some more bubbly. It was really cosy at Amanda's, we had nice music and we chatted for ages. We were all high with excitement about seeing each other again.

When we all decided we had had enough booze, we went upstairs to go to bed. She only had the one bedroom, but we all agreed to crash in her double bed. At this point there didn't seem anything in it. I've done this lots of times with other mates – I think it's a bit of a girlie thing.

We got into the bed together having stripped off to our undies. We started telling each other that we loved each other and had really missed not being together. We then were telling each other how nice our boobs were and nice bums, legs, eyes, lips etc. Then suddenly Sarah said she thinks I'm so fit and that if she were a bloke she would do this – with that she kissed me. I laughed, but she kept kissing me. I was very drunk and just thought, Oh well, and kissed her back. Amanda just pissed herself with laughing. When we looked up she had her video camera on us, so we kept kissing and playing up to the camera. It was all a bit of fun.

I stopped kissing Sarah and took the video camera and encouraged Amanda to kiss Sarah. I filmed them snogging. It wasn't really sexual. It was nice and we all enjoyed it.

It was good and felt nice but we didn't take it too seriously. It was a drunken thing to do. We all agreed to get rid of the evidence because if it got in the wrong hands it could be really embarrassing and none of us wanted to watch it again. We made a pact not to tell anyone (sorry, girls). But we do have the odd sarcastic joke between ourselves.

We never did anything more than kiss and cuddle and I don't feel tempted to do it again. I like men. Although I have had the odd dream involving girls, it's not by choice, it just sometimes happens.

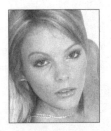

CHARLIE STORM

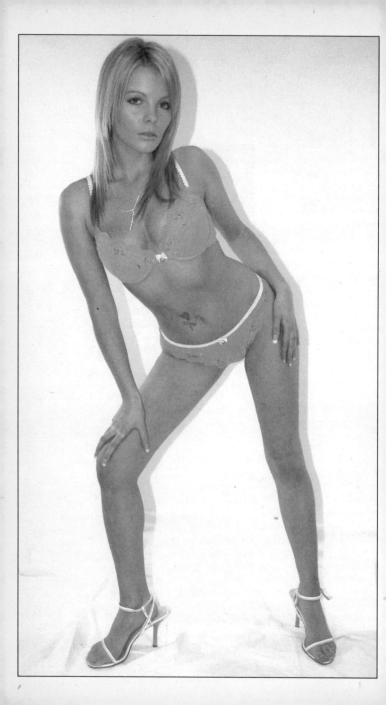

CHARLIE STORM

Name: Charlotte How
Model/Dance Name: Charlie Storm
Star Sign: Aries
Age: 22
Vital Stats: 34C-23-32
Lives: Gloucester /London
Fave Food: Dominos pizzas
Fave Drink: Water

Where do you work?
I am a full-time model, working around the UK and Europe, but have also done some assignments in Hollywood. I do regular appearances in the *Sport*, *Zoo* magazine and many more middle-shelf mags.

How did you get into modelling?
Each time I am asked this question I always

have to pinch myself, because I would never have thought that I would ever get to be a model.

When I was 11, I went to a school called St Teilos. This was a church school in Cardiff, South Wales. My mum had struggled to get me in there. But I attended confirmation classes and church on a regular basis. When you go to high school for the first time I think that almost every pupil in the first form gets picked on by the older ones at some point in their first year. When it came to me, I thought the bullying would not last long and all blow over quickly. I was wrong. Pupils were bullying me in my own year. It would always be over small things that others would find funny, but would really hurt me.

The girls would sit in the corridors with their legs straight out, stopping me from getting to my lessons. If I were passing girls on the stairs they would put their leg out to trip me up. When I was in my classes, I was afraid of putting my hand up for anything, as it would cause the bullying to get worse and they would call me names like 'Swot' or 'Teacher's Pet'.

I would also get pushed down the school stairs, get laughed at as I walked through the school and I would even get my lunch stolen.

I felt this bullying was all down to being ugly. I never told anyone about my problems and felt that telling on them would only make things worse. I felt like I had nobody to turn to and it made me very depressed. I would always say to my mum that I was ill so she wouldn't send me to school.

Eventually, it came to a point where I felt I was wasting my life and time at school. So I left as soon as I had the chance.

I was given the opportunity to work as an apprentice hairdresser in a salon, but after a year moved to another salon called Timba Hair Co, in Cardiff. I worked there for about six months before realising that hairdressing was not really for me. I moved around various jobs for a while trying to find something that I would enjoy, but didn't really find anything.

When I was 19 I needed extra cash, so took a job as a barmaid in a popular pub in Bridgend, called The Roof. It was a very busy pub that was popular with young people and regarded as the place to be on a night out.

It was good for me as the night would go very quickly and, as I was the other side of the bar, I would not be out spending my money. I would get chatted up a lot but thought that most guys were just drunk and after one thing.

There was a very good-looking guy that regularly came into the pub with his football teammates, he used to tease me a lot about not smiling while I worked, especially when I served him. He used to call me sexy and told me that I was far too good to be working in a bar and that I should be a model instead. I thought he was just taking the mickey, because I had always been called ugly in my school days. I eventually ended up going out with this guy; his name is Jason March and we are still together and very happy.

I did start doing modelling and couldn't believe that I was getting regular work. I was quite shocked one day when I had a phone call from a great and very talented photographer, Jens Wikholm, better known as Popstar. He was enquiring about my availability and willingness to travel to Majorca for a week with other models to do some shoots. It was to do a variety of shoots that were to be used in *ICE magazine*, either as content or more hopefully as a pullout supplement.

This was a hard decision to make as I had just moved to a new house, a lovely old cottage, and did have other work planned close to home. After talking it through with a few people, I rearranged my planned work and agreed to go.

My parents picked me up on a Sunday and drove me to Luton Airport. I never forget that moment as I didn't want to leave my little Labrador puppy (Diesel) behind, as I had only just bought him. Once at the airport, I met up with the other models and Phil (one of my agents). Jens was already over there. I felt a lot more relaxed at this point and it was taking my mind off Diesel.

The flight and travelling to the accommodation was not that long and it was bearable with the company I had. We arrived at this amazing villa that was in the middle of nowhere. It looked very posh and I couldn't wait to get to my room, making sure I was sharing with a friend I had made during the journey there.

Later that night, we all sat round the open log fire discussing what work we were going to be doing. This is where I had a shock ... they required me to be up at five in the morning to go to the beach for a sunrise picture set. I managed to get up and go but the weather was not at its best and I felt cold and tired all through the shoot. But I stuck with it and did my best. I knew that working in a bar or restaurant was not going to make me lots of money, nor was it going to get me any fame. I always wanted to be known for my achievements and not regretting 'what ifs' later on in my life.

This shoot gave me so much confidence. I knew I had the backing from my boyfriend so on my return I had no hesitation in giving up my regular work in the pursuit of happiness and success as a full-time model.

I jumped straight in the deep end and went full-time straight away. I took a big risk and it was very hard not having any money for most that things girls want at that age, clothes, make-up, CDs etc etc. I really did struggle from the start but the most important thing was that I had a home and food that my boyfriend paid for, in order to let me get on with my modelling career.

I started off by doing a lot of research on the internet about the industry, photographers, agencies and, most importantly, how to ensure my safety at all times. This is the biggest lesson I learned and always pass this on to other budding models that look for advice from me. I spent a lot of time with my boyfriend doing pics with a digital camera we had bought. This allowed me to learn all about my posing, make-up and clothing while giving me the odd pic or two that I could use for advertising myself on model-style websites.

I hadn't, at this point, got any appointments with agencies, because either due to my pics not being quite good enough, or the fact I felt slightly nervous in approaching them and being rejected. I also felt awkward asking my boyfriend or parents for money to travel, because I never knew if I would be able to give them it back.

I began to realise that I needed more money for clothing and travelling to get some pics done by a photographer to enable me to advertise my ability more and get into the good agencies. Unfortunately, I was finding that the photographers that were more than willing to help with pictures were really just interested in taking advantage of me.

I eventually got the confidence to send some pics off to the Sam Bond Model Agency and was surprised with the swift response I got. She liked my look and wanted me to go to her office ASAP for a face-to-face meeting. Unfortunately, I never made it to her office owing to my decision to take a year out, which I will explain later.

What's the biggest fee/tip you have ever earned?

A guy who wanted to do some video and pictures with me, along the theme of 'wet' once contacted me.

As you can imagine, I initially thought this might be something to do with wetting yourself ... however, when he explained it further, it merely involved me being fully clothed and getting wet in water, such as a bath, shower, stream etc. It sounded fairly straightforward and, considering he was offering to pay me £500 for a weekend's work, I agreed to go along with it.

As the date for the shoot got closer, the guy wanted to make the weekend work easier by staying in hotels/B&Bs for the Friday and Saturday nights so we could get early starts. I didn't mind this, but when he said his brother would also be there, I got slightly concerned, as I didn't know either one of them. I asked if he minded my boyfriend, Jas, coming along for my safety and he would pay his own way. He agreed to this.

We travelled on the Friday to a small B&B located in the Neath Valley (Wales), where we first met up with David and his brother. Another model was also supposed to join us for the weekend but failed to turn up. That night we had a few drinks and some food whilst getting to know what the weekend fully involved. At this point it did seem fairly straightforward and quick.

Saturday morning, we all walked (with equipment) to a very secluded waterfall. It was a cold day and the water looked even colder. I was starting to have second thoughts about doing this, but knew I couldn't let these people down now we had come this far. I had clothes provided, which were slightly old-fashioned and nothing that I would really want to be seen in. The clothes reminded me of what I would find in my granny's wardrobe! I kept thinking it was some kind of set-up.

CHARLIE STORM

It just seemed too easy. All I had to do was wear these clothes with no bra on so they became see-through as I moved around the water and waterfall, then remove them down to just my knickers. Thirty minutes later, I had done what they wanted for that day. It was hard building up the courage to get in the cold water but once I was in it was fairly OK. My feet turned blue and it took me absolutely ages to warm up, even with the help of extra clothing.

We finished the day's shoot at around noon and decided to travel to Tenby ready for the next day's shoot. Again, we stayed in a B&B that night ready for the next day. Sunday came and we got up early and travelled to a local farm, where we left the cars and walked down to a small, secluded beach. I felt more worried this day as the weather was not very good and the sea was rough. Plus, I couldn't swim! This was exactly the same as the previous day, old-fashioned clothing and rolling around in the water (surf) while being filmed. Except this time, as I was taking the clothes off, they were getting swept away very quickly and I was getting blasted by the sea and sand. Regardless of the weather, there were lots of people around watching the filming.

Sunday's shoot also took about 30 minutes and I was back home in bed by 4pm, £500 richer.

It was a very memorable experience and both David and his brother were great guys to work with. However, I did end up in bed for a few days afterwards with flu.

What highstreet publications have you been in?

The majority of my work is aimed at middle-shelf magazines. I have been published in quite a few so far including the *Daily Star* (Page 3), O2 Mobile phone video shoot (downloadable videos for your mobile), *Sport Girls* magazine, *Front* magazine (schoolgirl cover shoot), *Loaded* magazine, *News of the World* (Sex in the Office feature), the *Sport* (regular Page 3 and freebie advertising), *ICE* magazine (supplement, Babes in the Wood shoot in Spain and girlzone feature), *Zoo* magazine (cover), *Modified Drive* (online magazine), *Biker* (cover). I've also been doing TVX presenting and other website work.

I enjoy going on shoots and each is memorable, because each one is different in many ways. I enjoy working with different photographers and on different locations/studios. I take all my work seriously as I always want to produce great results that both the photographer and myself will be pleased with. I feel a great sense of achievement when my pictures are published, especially when they are covers.

CHARLIE STORM

What other work have you done?

Apart from my hairdressing apprenticeship and bar work, I have done work in LA or Hollywood. It was always a place that made me curious. I wanted to research how the glamour and adult industry worked over there. It is a place that you hear so much about in films and modelling and I was hooked.

I made a few contacts out there, which were willing to help with flights and accommodation and work if I wanted it. This was enough to get me packing and fly over there (with my boyfriend at my side for security).

While I was there, I was shown around some photographers that did some amazing pictures, compared to those I had seen in the UK. There was one person though that really stood out and impressed me. I was instantly inspired to work with this photographer before I returned home to the UK. All I knew at this point was her name was Suze Randell and she worked out of LA. I asked my contact to take me to see her, if she would allow it. I desperately wanted her to shoot me, but was also keen just to meet her if she wasn't interested in shooting me.

My contact showed Suze a few of my photos. Great news, she was very keen to meet me and possibly work with me. The day came for my shoot and I was really nervous. I didn't know what to expect. When we arrived at the studio, it was a big garage-type business unit in a quiet back street. It was not what I expected from the glamorous photos I had seen. However, once inside, I was gobsmacked at the set that was being built and the whole camera/lighting set-up. There were a lot of people about and they made both of us feel very welcome and special.

The set looked very expensive and was surely designed for a famous model. Without having time to think any further, I was introduced to the make-up artist and fashion stylist, who were so nice to me, spending hours altering clothes and making me up for the perfect set I had seen being built earlier.

Suze had made me look and feel like a princess and brought out a confidence that I never knew I had. After an hour or two of shooting, a small camera crew came into the studio to conduct an interview with Suze. They asked if I would be willing to be part of it, and, not knowing what it was about or where it was going to be screened, I agreed. I later found out that the crew was actually from the UK and worked for the BBC. It was for a documentary on the growing adult industry and was called Sex Empires. It did get screened in the UK on BBC2 and I was featured on it while Suze was taking pictures of me. This whole day was something I could never have dreamed of prior to going to LA and I will always remember it and, more so, my whole experience of working with probably one of the best photographers in the world.

The work I did with Suze Randell might have been adult and above the level that I ever wanted to go to, but I found it more glamorous than middle-shelf and it was very easy money. However, the work itself wasn't rewarding enough for me, compared to achieving middle-shelf work in the UK.

I like a challenge and wanted to be seen on magazine covers, so Hollywood was a 'no-no' for me, so I returned to the UK. I'm now just doing what I love best, but Suze Randell is someone who I will always remember and look up to. All her work is a masterpiece.

Do you have any famous friends?
I hang out at a lot of London clubs that celebrities go to, such as Penthouse Club, Embassy, Ten Rooms etc. I mainly mix with other models and photographers when I'm out, but you're always amongst popstars and actors. It's a lot better atmosphere in these places compared to your usual nightclub that's full of

drunk guys coming on to you, with all the regular cheesy chat-up lines and girls that are bitchy towards you for no real reason. Being around people like yourself is more relaxing, allowing you to enjoy the night. It also feels great not having to queue to get in anywhere.

What does your family think of the work you do?
I didn't really tell my family for a long time, as I was slightly concerned about what they would say or do. I eventually talked to my mum about it and she was very good about the whole thing. But I didn't tell my dad for a while after, as I didn't know which way he would take it.

One day I decided to just bite the bullet and come out with it, although this was easier said than done. I actually told him one day, but just said I was doing clothed modelling. He was OK about this. The following week I decided to tell him I was now doing underwear work. Again he was fairly OK with it. He was just a bit concerned about my safety. The pattern continued week by week, until it got to the glamour/nude part. I was shitting myself at this point. I prepared myself for the worst. However, he shocked the hell out of me. My dad was very supportive of what I had chosen to do.

I, personally, don't feel that, deep down, either of my parents are happy with my chosen work.

CHARLIE STORM

It didn't take long for the rest of the family to know what I was up to, including my sisters who, at first, took great pleasure in taking the mickey out of me. Then, when I was published in a magazine, my sisters actually took more interest in what I was doing and started bragging to friends and work colleagues about me.

I don't think anyone from school knows what I do as I don't use my real name in my work.

What's your funniest moment?

There was one night; I was out at the Embassy Club, at one of my agency parties (SuperModel). As always I was enjoying myself, dancing and having a few drinks. I usually know what I'm doing the majority of the time but that night I really didn't have a clue. I was out with a few people from *ICE* magazine (Jens the photographer who I mentioned previously was there). It was a great night in the club, with many models and celebrities enjoying the atmosphere. Towards the end of the night we stayed in the VIP section of the club, taking advantage of the free drinks, courtesy of SuperModel Agency. When we left the club we were heading off towards Stringfellows to enjoy the last hours of our night out. But then I saw flashing and heard my name being shouted out by over 20 tabloid photographers. As I was a little tipsy I decided to quickly flash my boobs and walk away. Then I thought hang on a min; I best make the most of this to get in the papers. I quickly bent over and flashed my bum while hanging on to the railings outside the club. The bouncer then grabbed me and said, 'Not outside the club', and moved me along. The tabloids followed me and shouted for me to get on the police car that was parked up. Again, being drunk and knowing it would get me some publicity in the papers, I bent over the police car flashing my bum and boobs at the cameras. Everyone that was with me was shocked and tried pulling me off the car. They said I was lucky I wasn't arrested. But I managed not to get arrested and ended up in Stringfellows as planned. I didn't remember anything that had happened, until I was told a week later by one of the people from *ICE* magazine. They said it was in the *Daily Star*. I didn't know whether to laugh or cry. Alcoholic memory is always a bit dangerous, but I guess I got some exposure out of it – that's the main thing!

What's your scariest moment?

I was booked for a shoot that involved an early start, so me and my boyfriend were booked into a B&B, which I think was called The Swan, in

CHARLIE STORM

Bath. It was a very old pub that was once a quarry house. The room was all stone with uneven floorboards that made you feel like you were sliding out of the bed when trying to sleep.

We had some food and a few drinks that night which helped us get to sleep very quickly. But, in the middle of the night I was woken up by the sound of banging above our room. I opened my eyes but it was absolutely pitch black, I couldn't even see my hand right in front of my face. The banging stopped, but I still felt scared being awake on my own and not being able to see anything! Then, all of a sudden, I could hear the floorboards moving in a pattern of someone walking in the room from the door right up to my bed. I was so scared I couldn't move. I just lay there waiting for something to happen. Nothing did happen, apart from the banging, which started above the room again. I was too afraid to wake my boyfriend up and spent the rest of the night under the covers unable to sleep.

The next morning at breakfast, I asked the landlord about the room above us, to which he replied, 'There are no rooms above yours, just the attic.' This made me feel worse, especially when he said other people had told him about various noises.

My shoot did not go too well that day owing

to the lack of sleep and the fact that I couldn't stop thinking about the noises. I will never forget that night and will definitely not be going back to that pub.

Have you ever turned down work and why?
I have turned down a lot of work. The majority of offers have being requests for adult work, or perverted people that want to get off while they photograph you. But I never turn down middle-shelf work as this raises your profile and who knows when your next shoot might be. The modelling industry changes from time to time and most photographers get their castings done at the beginning of the year to get all their models for the year.

I do bondage work, which some people class as porn, but I'm always clothed when I do it, so I don't see what the big deal is. My limit is posing full-frontal nude, which is mostly required in the likes of *ICE* and *Front* etc.

Do you have a sexual fantasy?
I do have a fantasy that involves me and another girl experimenting with sex, while being secretly watched! When I'm out with model friends I sometimes snog them as it gives us both attention and publicity in the papers. I don't go any further

than kissing. If I went further it would only end up in a porn magazine! Tabloids give more publicity than porn magazines, so it really wouldn't be worth going any further. Plus, I don't get paid for it. I will only do this kind of thing when it's worth it, like if a photographer walks past etc. I do enjoy it. It's great fun.

What's your most memorable sexual experience?

I read in a magazine that making homemade porn movies can help improve a relationship. So one day I decided to go digging around the house looking to find Jas's porn films. I knew he'd have some somewhere, like every other guy does, right? Wrong, Jas didn't have any!

I decided to ask Jas if he could get any porn videos. 'Yes, but what do you want one for?' he asked, with a big grin on his face. I told him I thought it would be fun to watch one together. After a few days, he came home with a few, saying I had a choice. For one reason or another we never got to watch them together, but while he was at work I got curious and watched them. Not for pervy reasons, I just wanted to get an idea on how to make one.

Nervously I had dug out the camcorder and did a bit of experimenting. Because there was no pressure on me to perform in front of anyone, I got on OK. I experimented for a few days to get a bit of confidence and eventually I built up to a proper scene involving me stripping off and having a little bit of fun on the bed. I was really excited doing the video, but couldn't bring myself to watch it.

After a few weeks I plucked up the courage to show my boyfriend. He came home from playing football and I put the tape in his hand. He smiled and said, 'What is it?' I said, 'Just play it and you'll find out.' He did, but I couldn't sit there and watch it with him so I ran upstairs, bright red. After about 20 minutes he came upstairs looking all shocked. He was very horny and I was well impressed that it had worked!

After a mind-blowing sex session, I asked him if we could make one together. He agreed. I spent a long time setting the room, lining up the camera and sorting out the music.

It went really well and was easier than I thought, plus it made sex much more fun. Now my boyfriend watches my own porn films instead of other people's – I just wish I could take it to the next step and make one for him with another girl.

What do you think about group sex? Have you tried it?

I would definitely love to experiment with another girl alone, or with my partner just watching. I don't fancy girls but it's fun to experiment with sex. If you don't try it, you'll never know. I also fool around with girls to make guys jealous. I think I'm a bit of a tease at times and like the attention. I have never had a threesome but I would be up for it if I could trust the girl and she was happy to do it secretly without anyone knowing about it. I'm up for trying almost anything to do with sex; I just love to try new things. I did once think about taking things a step further on the girl thing. I browsed a few websites and talked to many girls through email and chat. Jas did warn me about the possible problems with doing this, but I liked it. I even found one girl that sounded exactly what I wanted. Well, that was until I found out it was a guy! You have to be so careful these days. This has probably scared me away from finding a girl this way, but I don't know how else I could find someone and to make sure that it was safe and anonymous. It not the kind of thing you can just ask your mates, is it?

What advice would you give to someone who wanted to get into this business?

Get yourself a good agent. I made work harder for myself because I didn't have an agent and felt I didn't need one. I even turned agents away. Top agents never guarantee you work, but they're always there to give you honest advice and have regular clients they trust, which means you are a lot safer in the industry as there are, as I know, some very strange people out there.

Which bloke do you fancy the most?
Umm ... guess it would have to be Nigel Harmen from *EastEnders*.

Tell me a secret ··· During my career I decided to take some time out of my work, and take time to evaluate where I actually wanted to go with my career. Well, that's what I told everyone and that's what they have all thought, until now.

The truth behind this time out was I discovered I was pregnant and I had to go through a problematic abortion. When I first fell pregnant I was totally devastated. I felt like it was the end of the world for me. I was working as a model and everything was going really well for me. I had an appointment with Sam Bond, a top agency for glamour models.

Then I started to break out in spots and I got itchy skin when I put on moisturiser or self-tan. I would have bad hair days, regardless of what shampoo I used. It started to really depress me. I remember thinking to myself, What the hell is going on? Then I started to put on a little bit of weight. I thought, How can I be? I'm eating the same regular food as I always do. I also started to find that I could hardly stay awake through the day. I called the doctor for some advice, but ended up speaking to one of the nurses. I told her all about the way I was feeling and the symptoms I was having. She said, 'I think you need to get a pregnancy test.' I was in shock. I didn't know what to say. It had never crossed my mind that it could be this.

As soon as I put the phone down, I got my coat on and dashed out the door and into town. I finally ended up at a chemist, but it took me ages to build myself up to buy a pregnancy kit. I hurried to the nearest public toilet and tested myself straight away. It came up positive. I was pregnant! I couldn't believe it. So I went to another chemist. This time I bought three tests to take home. Over the course of that week, I tested myself at different times of the day. It made no difference; they all came up POSITIVE!

I was feeling so sad and didn't know how to tell Jas. When I eventually built up the courage to tell him, he was devastated. Jas didn't want a baby in his life at that time and nor did I as my career was just starting. When we both agreed that it was the wrong time to start a family, I made the call to my doctor for an appointment.

I got an appointment the next day and discussed the situation with my doctor. I explained that I wanted to get rid of it ASAP. The doctor asked, 'Can't you keep it?' I explained about my career and how it would affect me. He replied, 'You have plenty of time for that.' He didn't understand, but I insisted that I was having none of it. He said I would possibly lose my sex drive and it could cause me depression. I really didn't give a shit at this point and thought, Yeah, whatever, as if it's gonna come to that!

I had a follow-up appointment at the hospital and, again, the nurses and doctor tried to talk me out of my decision. Yet again I was told about the possible side-effects of low sex drive and depression. But I was not really listening. I had my abortion booked for two days later. As a lot of people, like family and friends are against this kind of thing, Jas and I decided to keep it a secret and no one was ever going to know.

The problem was I really couldn't keep it to myself for some reason and the next day I did tell my sister. She's really cool and I trusted her not to say anything. I also asked her if she would come along with me, as – this may sound really bad – Jas went to play football the day of my abortion so his friends wouldn't suspect anything. He has never missed a day of football since he had started going; even when he was injured he would go to watch. Prior to Jas going to the football match, he dropped my sis and me to the hospital in Llantrisant. He came with us to the ward, but left soon after and said, 'I will come and see you as soon as I have finished.'

I had a private room, but couldn't believe the hospital had put me in the maternity area! The nurses gave me a bathrobe and inserted some tablets inside me. I filled in lots of forms, giving them consent to cremate the foetus. I was so mixed up and really didn't know what I was doing for the best.

I was too far gone, 16 weeks, to have this abortion done the usual way, so I had to actually give birth to it, but it would be dead. I was told to lie there and wait until I start to bleed. It took about 30 minutes from when I had the tablets inserted. I was in the worst pain ever, 50 times worse than your worst-ever period pain. It was terrible.

It went on for about three hours non-stop. All I was given were painkillers to help with the pain, but they did nothing for me. I was in so much pain, so much so that my sister neglected me, as she couldn't stand it. She just stormed out of the room. It hurt that she left me there alone, but I didn't blame her. I might have done the same in her situation. I started to cry because I was left alone. I was in so much pain and didn't know what the hell was happening.

Jas eventually turned up about an hour later. I don't know whether I felt happy to see him, or angry because he had left me! He went white when he saw me and I remember him saying, 'Are you OK?' all the time. I wanted to say, 'What the f*** do you think?' but I couldn't, as I sensed that he felt very guilty for not being there.

I was sitting on the toilet in my room bleeding non-stop, when I had this unbelievable pain in my lower stomach and I couldn't move. While Jas went for the nurse, I heard a splash. The foetus had come out. The nurse arrived and shouted, 'Don't look.' But I couldn't stop myself looking. It was so tiny and everything seemed to be there, I really never ever expected it to be like that. I hadn't thought of it as a baby until that point. I felt guilty, but deep down I still knew that it was the right choice. The nurse removed it and took it out of the room. I got back into my bed.

About 20 minutes after it had arrived the pain started to fade and everything was nearly over. The doctor and nurses came to see me and did a few tests etc. A further three or four hours later the hospital was happy to let me go home. I felt a bit better but not great. I was given antibiotics to take for a week to keep away infections in the womb. As you can imagine, I really didn't feel like working straight away and thought I would take a few weeks off.

I spent most of my time relaxing, watching daytime TV and sleeping. I was slightly bored and a few weeks went by before I started to snap at Jas. He would come home from work and I would shout at him, blaming him for everything. It would start over silly things such as leaving the freezer door open while cooking and always end up, somehow, with the abortion.

Days turned into weeks and I was still blaming him for silly things, turning it into a hate campaign against him. I really don't know how he put up with it! I think any other guy would have just left me.

My mum would also phone (still not knowing what I had done) just to see how I was and I would snap at the simplest things she would say. I would say very hurtful things to her, not thinking or knowing what I was doing. It was the same for anyone in my family, even my sister who had been there with me. I didn't want to go out of the house nor did I really want to stay in. I was going mad with too much time to think about what had happened.

A few months went by and Jas and I did start having a few better moments. I felt as if I was starting to control myself a little better, until one day he said to me, 'You haven't wanted any sex since ...' I shouted before he could finish his sentence, 'I hate sex!' I was back in my hatred moody mode. He said, 'You have always liked sex.' He was right; I had enjoyed sex with him before I had this. Any time we had the slightest argument I would just walk off making the rowing get worse, plus I would still be blaming him for anything and everything. Any time I heard sex on the TV or radio or if Jas mentioned the word sex, it made me feel sick.

I then started to think back to what the doctor and nurses had told me about losing my sex drive. This started to make me feel worse; I didn't want sex and felt that Jas would go off with someone else because I wasn't having any with him. What could I do? My mum kept going on at me, asking if everything was ok. Again, I would just snap at her. She knew I wasn't telling her something.

I eventually started to get myself together and would have sex with Jas, but I was not as adventurous as before and would put little or no effort into it, just lying there. Not the nicest thing in the world for Jas.

I began to get more and more depressed and lost confidence in myself. I would even cover up my body when I went to bed and would cover up any time Jas was about. I would burst into tears for no reason, no matter where we were. I would also say to Jas, if we went out in the car, 'I don't want to die, I'm scared of going out in the car. Can I stay home?' For some reason I was afraid of dying. It was depressing him; I was bringing up all these morbid things and could never feel safe wherever I went. I even turned to Jas one day, during an argument, 'It's all your fault because you made me get rid of my baby.' His face dropped ... he went silent for what seemed an eternity. I really didn't understand what I had said. He spoke to me afterwards and said, 'It was both our choice, not just one of us who wanted to get rid of it.'

It just seemed to go on and on, not getting any better. I wanted my baby back. I felt like someone had stolen it from me. I was heart-broken and Jas was to blame for it and everything else.

It came to a big head one day when my mum was over at our house visiting. As usual something petty caused me to snap at Jas and my mum couldn't believe it. She was gobsmacked at the way I was being, but Jas stood up to my mum very bravely and said, 'She had an abortion a few months ago and she hasn't been the same since and I don't know what to do any more.' My mum was devastated. She turned to me and said, 'What the hell did you get rid of it for?' I started to cry and said, 'I don't know but I want it back.' She immediately threw her arms around me. I didn't think she would stand by me, but she did. I knew, and she knew, I had made a mistake, but none of us had the power to turn back the clock. My dad was also understanding when we told him. I really did fear telling them, not knowing what they would have said or done. If I had known they were going to be like this, then I suppose I would have confided in them previously.

My parents really helped me get through some of the bad times; they would take me out rather than me being in the house dwelling on the past. Jas had a full-time job, so it was awkward for him.

During the whole episode I know I was very selfish, just thinking about myself, how it affected *me* and what I wanted. Not even once did I ask Jas about his side of things. I never gave him the opportunity to tell me how he was feeling. Then, finally, one day Jas said to me he regretted getting rid of it too. It just felt like the best option at the time for us both.

He had stood by me through the whole thing. I would cry each night; even baby adverts would make me cry. That's how heart-broken I was. I completely forgot about my modelling career for months.

I gradually started to get my life back on track. Jas helped me to get my confidence back. It took time and a lot of effort but it did get better and I eventually took the big step of going back to work. I spent time following the industry and missing what I could have been doing. I watched the progress of models and knew that I would have been at that stage if I had put the effort in. Towards the end of the year, I made a big effort to get back into the modelling and achieve what I had initially wanted. This is when I re-contacted Sam Bond.

I still cry some nights and talking about this now has put a big pain in my heart. This has been hard to do but I'm looking ahead now and want people to take my advice – before you do what I did, talk to people (family, friends or doctors) because they may help in ways you never thought they would. I would not recommend to anyone to go though with something like this without fully exploring all the consequences, as you will regret it ... forever! Even if you feel like you wouldn't at the time, your hormones kick in and change how you feel. I have to live with my decision for the rest of my life and it hurts.

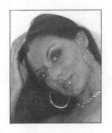

DANI

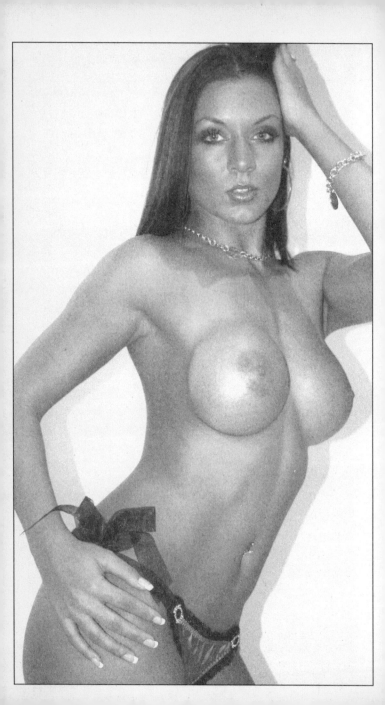

DANI

Name: Dani Thompson
Model/Dance Name: Dani
Star Sign: Leo
Age: 21
Vital Stats: 32DD-26-32
Lives: Norwich
Fave Food: Prawn Cocktail
Fave Drink: Champagne & cocktails

Where do you work?

I currently work at Devils Advocate, which is a lap-dancing club in Norwich. I have been working there for nearly a year. I have also worked at another club in the area called Angels in Great Yarmouth.

I enjoy dancing, but really want to make a career out of my modelling. It's still early days, but I have managed to get in quite a few highstreet magazines, such as *Max Power*, *Nuts*, *Daily Sport* and in the *Loaded* Ultimate Showgirls Competition.

I'm really trying to push the modelling side of my career at the moment and have just set up my own website, www.dani-model.co.uk, which is proving very successful

How did you get into modelling?

I began working as a lap-dancer because I needed some cash. I was 20 at the time and had heard that you could earn good money lap-dancing. I called a club in Great Yarmouth called Angels and I was invited to an audition. The audition was the worst part, as I had to audition in front of two other girls, who were head dancers at the time. They were really good dancers, so the pressure was on. I must have done OK, 'cause I got the job and started the next night. I worked at the club for a while, as it was a quiet club and it gave me time to learn how to do lots of tricks on the pole. When I felt comfortable about my routines I started getting itchy feet and wanting to move on to somewhere bigger. I didn't really get on with the house mum at Angels at the time and she started cutting my shifts. I was really pissed off with it all so I left. I called the club that I work in now, Devils Advocate in Norwich, and got an audition on the same night that I quit. I auditioned on stage in front of a full club and started there that very night.

I also started modelling at the age of 20, after working with a friend, who was a photographer. I decided to try and put together a portfolio and started to work for a few different photographers to build up different styles of photographs.

I don't know when it was that I started to want to be a model, it just happened. Without trying to sound big-headed, I found that men were always interested in me and thought I would take advantage of my assets. It also came at a good time, as I was having a few family problems and needed the money to be able to take care of myself.

What's the biggest fee/tip you have ever earned?

I was once paid £600 just to talk to a guy. He had been going out with a lap-dancer in London and was really depressed that they had split up. He didn't want me to dance for him; he just wanted to talk. I wasn't even listening to most of the conversation, just nodding my head and saying 'yes' every now and then in a sympathetic way, to make it look like I was listening! What a shock I got when he handed over £600 and thanked me for listening.

TELL ME A SECRET

Have you danced for any famous people?
Have you been in any highstreet publications?
I haven't danced for anyone famous that I know of, but I don't always pay too much attention to the guys in the club, so maybe I have. I have been in quite a few magazines such as *Max Power* magazine, *Nuts*, *Fast Car*, *Loaded* etc.

What other work have you done?
Before I started dancing I worked as a buyer's assistant, but found that I could earn more money from modelling and dancing. But at the same time I am a realist, so I am also currently at college in Great Yarmouth and studying for my HND in fashion and textiles. It is my last year and I'm working on my final collection on design and clothes making. I have based my collection on showgirls.

I am taking a year out in 2005 to concentrate on my modelling career, which I'm hoping will take off. If my modelling career doesn't take off, then I will concentrate on a career in design and probably have my own boutique. But then again, if I do become a successful model, I may still open up my own designer boutique, but charge more for the clothes!

DANI

Do you have any famous friends?

My best friend is Kerri Parker, who is a well-known glamour model. I met her through a photographer. We get on great together and every time we are out, whether shopping or partying, we have a great laugh, we have had many funny experiences together. I remember the day she won Max Star Babe at the *Max Power* Car Show and we were suppose to be driving home to Norwich from Birmingham. What a nightmare – now I do go on about guys saying things that girls can't do, like map reading etc. but, guys, I have to agree with you on this one. I really can't read maps. I ended up directing us to Manchester, which was the total opposite direction. What a dizz.

The best party we have been to together was a Bond theme night at one of the clubs in Norwich. We went dressed up in bikinis. Kerri went as the Ursula Andress Bond girl in a white bikini and I went as Halle Berry in an orange bikini. We were the least-dressed girls in the club, so that meant we were plied with free Champagne in the VIP lounge all night long. After about four bottles, we were well drunk. If that wasn't bad enough, to make matters more embarrassing, my friend, Mark, filmed me on his videophone. I now have to bribe him with free dances when he comes to the club just so that he doesn't show anyone!

What does your family think of the work you do?

My mum doesn't really mind what I do. I think she would prefer it if I had a 'normal' job. But she keeps all of my magazine cutouts in a scrapbook, so I think secretly that she is really proud. When I first told my mum that I was working in a lap-dancing bar, she didn't really understand what it entailed. It was only when I had a necklace on that said 'stripper', that her boyfriend said, 'That's a nasty business, you don't want to get into that.' I turned to him and said, 'What do you think I do when I go to work?' Once she got over the shock, she started being OK with it.

Since I started to work in the club I have seen so many people I know, ex-boyfriends, people from school, people I have worked with. Most of my friends were shocked at first, but none of them was jealous and they often come in for a drink. I have also met some really good friends at the club.

What's your funniest moment?

I'm really lucky I guess, because my life is full of funny moments. Kerri Parker's 21st birthday party at Brannigans was a hoot – it was pimps and bunnies. Although the time at the Bond theme night has to be one of the best. I was really drunk and fell down some stairs and lost the top of my bikini.

Then only last week me and my friend, Charlene, did a stag show at a rugby club. We stripped and whipped the stag and covered each other in whipped cream and licked it off. By the end of the show we were totally covered in the stuff! Mmmm, funny and ever-so-slightly pervy!

What's your scariest moment?

I haven't really got any scary moments as such. I am always really careful about where I go and I usually take someone with me, unless I know the photographer. I have had a few weird emails from men who have emailed me through my site telling me what they'd like to do to me, which I find a bit strange, seeing as they have never met me. I do have one scary moment, which is connected to another fun time I had. It was at a *Max Power* after-party in London. Yet again I got very drunk and I am missing about three hours of my life. I think I ended up in The Elysium VIP, but who knows? Very scary.

Have you ever turned down work and why?

I have had offers to do porn and nasty knickers-off, legs-open pictures. But I'm not interested in that line of modelling, so I have turned them all down. I am only looking to get into the classy end of the glamour business, like Jordan.

TELL ME A SECRET

Do you have a sexual fantasy?
It is not a unique fantasy. I would love to make love under a waterfall on a tropical island. Maybe with Orlando Bloom or David Beckham, or even Adam Garcia from *Coyote Ugly* – I'm not really fussed as long as it's a waterfall and it's with someone I want to be with.

What's your most memorable sexual experience?
I guess it would have to be just after my now ex-boyfriend proposed to me in Barcelona. I was quite drunk at the time and we went back to our room with a bottle of Champagne. I had bought some crotchless knickers to surprise him. I put them on while he was out of the room and waited on the bed for him. When he came back I could tell that he liked what he saw and he poured the Champagne everywhere and licked it off – mmm, very memorable.

What do you think about group sex? Have you tried it?
I have never tried it and probably never would. But hey, never say never!

What advice would you give to someone who wanted to get into the business?
Definitely do it and have fun!

DANI

Which bloke do you fancy the most?
Orlando Bloom

Tell me a secret ... I don't really have many secrets, but there is one that I have never told anyone. It was with my long-term boyfriend, Adam. We split up recently after being together for five years, since I was 16. When I was 17, we were at the stage where we were still exploring each other sexually.

Adam didn't live at home, which was a good thing, as his parents never liked me. I never used to go to his parents' home. However, one time they were out of the country on a skiing holiday and we thought it would be a good opportunity to go round and have the house to ourselves.

It was great. We snuggled up on the sofa and had a few drinks. When we were a bit tipsy, we started getting a bit frisky. Adam mentioned that his parents had a video camera and wouldn't it be a good idea to film us having sex.

As Adam didn't have a bedroom of his own at his parents, we decided to take advantage of theirs. After all it was a nice big bed and had much more room to produce good footage.

I will leave it up to your imagination as to what we got up to, but needless to say we had a good time.

I had to leave not long after and assumed that he would take the tape out and hide it. We didn't talk about it for ages after, but, when we did, I found to my horror that he hadn't taken it out. He had forgotten. His parents had been home for a while at this point, so too late to go and rescue it.

To this day I don't know what happened to it. I don't know whether his parents saw it or not. All I do know is no one has ever mentioned it. I'm hoping that, if they did find it, they just destroyed it when they found out what it was.

If it hasn't been destroyed then look out for it when I'm a famous model. It might be worth a few quid and worth selling, in a 'Paris Hilton/Pamela Anderson'-style moneymaking scheme!

I am a lot more careful now about what I get up to and where, and I particularly do not encourage video evidence!

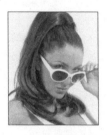

MADISON

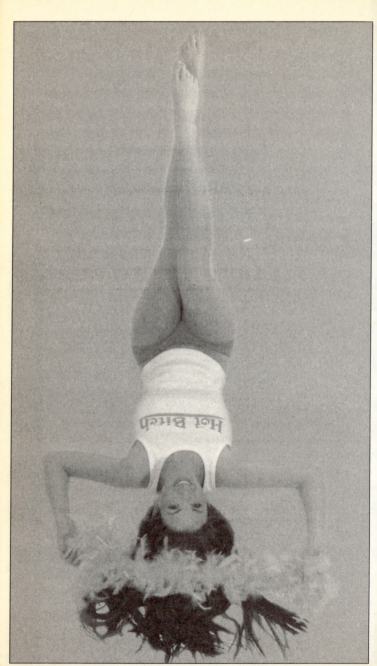

Photo © Starlight Photographics

MADISON

Name: Laura-Marie Apter
Model/Dance Name: Madison
Star Sign: Aries
Age: 23
Vital Stats: 34DD-24-34
Lives: The Wirral, North West
Fave Food: Chocolate
Fave Drink: Baileys

Where do you work?
I am a freelance model and travel to wherever the work is. I went to Lithuania in September 2004 to represent Great Britain in Miss Tourism Europe.

I started off being a glamour model, you know typical middle-shelf stuff and got a few small assignments before, and after, getting a breast enlargement. I saw how sleazy that side of the industry was and I got out. I believe that a girl can be glamorous without looking sleazy, so I am currently concentrating on my career in a different direction.

The first work that I got in my new career direction was doing a bit of charity work, catwalk and bridal fayres as well as beauty pageants. I have also been asked to enter Miss Planet in June 2005, which will be held in Greece

How did you get into modelling?

I first began modelling when I was 11. I attended a few modelling courses and, after graduating with an A*, things just progressed from there and I began doing fashion shows and bridal fayres

My first job was for Champagne and Roses, a bridal show in Ellesmere Port. It wasn't so much a big break, but good experience. I have never just relied on any agencies to get me work, because I think to be successful you have to push yourself. All the main assignments I have done have been because I have contacted companies directly and I try to make contacts through each job I do – it's all about networking.

What's the biggest fee/tip you have ever earned?

I was asked to go on a job in Peru at the end of January and would be paid £2,500. I'm not a very materialistic person and it's not about the money so I declined the offer and stayed at home to study for my exams.

What other work have you done?
I am currently studying anatomy and physiology so I can get into aromatherapy and massage. I'd eventually like to specialise in baby massage because I love children. I also do the occasional make-up job. (I'm a qualified make-up artist and have won a few national competitions over the past few years.)

What highstreet publications have you been in?
The first newspaper I was in was the *Sun* newspaper, modelling fashion clothes for Topshop and Miss Selfridge. I have since been in all my local papers and the *Daily Mirror*, plus *Fast Car*, *Max Power* etc. I have been asked to model for *Playboy*, but that's not my thing. I don't do adult stuff.

Do you have any famous friends?
I was invited to a party at Richard Branson's mansion in London last year and I was also invited to fly over to America to one of Hugh Hefner's famous Bunny Girl parties. I didn't end up going to America because I was a bit afraid of attending on my own. I have met quite a few

famous people when I do my pageants. I met Blue, Jordan, Lucy Pinder, Michelle Marsh, Dean Gaffney.

I have a friend who won *Model Behaviour*, which was a TV programme on Channel 4, a couple of years ago. They had two series and she was in the second. Camilla Priest is also a friend. She is from Sunderland and travels the world now and models for Christian Dior, Morgan, Faith and loads of other big companies. She is so lovely and she deserved to win the show more than any other model I know. So all my celeb dos comes from her. She went to Jay Z and Beyonce's London party last year and met them. She met Darius as well as Mario Testini (who did a photoshoot with her). Dolce and Gabanna, Chaka Khan, Christian Dior, too many too mention. Plus Nathan, the guy who was joint winner of the show and who was going out with Lady Victoria Hervey.

What does your family think of the work you do?
When I was wondering whether to be a topless model or not, I decided to give it a quick try. I didn't do it professionally though but I did phone the *Daily Mirror* and ask if they wanted to do an article on me and my mum's opinion regarding my modelling. They did. They paid my mum and

me £300 to go to London, plus travelling expenses. We were there for about an hour to have a couple of photos taken. They used a headshot of me and it looked like I never had a top on. So they put, 'My daughter is a topless model', and got my mum's opinions and mine.

My mum, dad, granddad and his wife and my boyfriend all support me in whatever I do as long as I'm happy. My brother gets embarrassed though, because some of his friends make jokes about me modelling. He's only 18, which is a critical age to be seen and be cool, so he's too busy trying to fit in with everyone

What's your funniest moment?

I used to do a lot of salsa dancing when I lived in Newcastle-upon-Tyne. I was dancing on a stage one night with my ex-boyfriend for Salsa Viva, my friend's business that became really popular in Newcastle. Tyne Tees Television were filming us and somebody put their drink on the stage. It got knocked over and I went flying on my bum down the steps. Luckily they never showed that clip, but I still watch *You've Been Framed* hoping that I won't appear on it!

What's your scariest moment?

I'm very careful about the work I choose to do, so

there hasn't really been a 'Scary Moment'. I was very nervous when I went to Lithuania. I had to sing our national anthem in front of the President, ambassadors, Lithuanian media and about 300 other people and – I must admit – I'm not the best of singers

Have you ever turned down work and why?
I have turned down so much work … *Playboy, Men and Motors*, work abroad. I don't do adult stuff and I like to feel comfortable about a job. If I'm not sure about an assignment, I won't do it. Simple as …

Do you have a sexual fantasy?
My sexual fantasy? Mmm, well actually, I have a few and they're all of me and my boyfriend. Firstly it would be to make love under the stars on the beach, with the water splashing on our feet. The next would be to have mad sex in the middle of a field in a wild storm with thunder and lightning and loads of rain. The final one is to have sex in a public place, the risk of being caught would just add to the thrill. I am definitely going to live all of these fantasies out!

What's your most memorable sexual encounter?
I haven't actually had many boyfriends but I do

intend to stay with my current boyfriend. We have the best sex. He's a Sagittarius and I'm an Aries and because we are both fire signs we are totally sexually compatible. The most memorable sexual encounter I had was the first time we made love – it was so intense.

What do you think about group sex? Have you tried it?
Each to their own, but I haven't tried it. I get quite jealous and I like to have all the attention.

What advice would you give to someone who wanted to get into this business?
In the modelling industry you always have to be careful, whether you're doing glamour or just fashion. There are always people waiting to take advantage of you in one way or another and that includes friends, agencies and photographers!

If you feel even slightly uncomfortable around anyone, try to distance yourself. If the photographer seems to be a bit sleazy, go with your gut instinct and find another photographer. You will feel more relaxed and your photos will turn out better. Always let someone know where you are. Keep a diary of assignments and get as many details of the job and contact person as possible. Always have credit on your mobile.

TELL ME A SECRET

Which bloke do you fancy the most?
My fella!!

Tell me a secret ... The main thing that people don't know about me is that, although I seem very confident, I am actually very insecure. I must get on my boyfriend's nerves because I need constant reassurance. I had my breasts enhanced in January 2004, but they took me to the wrong size (34FF), so I am currently saving to get them redone to a more 'normal'-looking size of 34DD. I am constantly thinking of ways to improve myself. I believe God gave us our bodies to work on, like an artist is given a blank canvas.

I suppose it seems a strange career to go into being as insecure as I am, but I love modelling. I believe the reason I am breaking away from the traditional glamour modelling is the way people treat you. They think that, because you look sexy and show a bit more of your body than the normal girl on the street, you are easy and a slag. That's not the attention I want. I like performing to an audience, but an audience that respects me as an individual.

The time when I felt the most self-conscious was at the Donny Show in Doncaster, South Yorkshire. I was giving out leaflets on 'How to win a new car'. It was probably the worst job I've ever done. I had to wear a sexy police uniform and it was raining. I wasn't covered up much because the outfit was very skimpy and I kept getting lecherous men walking past and groping me. OK, I accept that the idea was that I got attention but it was just the way they were looking at me that gave me the creeps. I bet every single one of them had a girlfriend or wife. I wonder how they would feel if their partner was treated like that.

It was a long day. I was freezing cold and I had to put up with these ignorant men, who probably believed it was OK to treat me like a piece of meat, because of the way I was dressed. I could have easily walked out after five minutes, but I am professional and I had made a commitment to do the job. I doubt very much that I'll be working at that show, or similar shows, ever again.

Apart from the bad experience at the Donny Show, I've had guys talking to my chest because they're showing off in front of their friends, grabbing my arse and even attempting to grab my boobs. How dare they?! Guys think that, because a girl does modelling and has a large chest, she must be totally dizzy and enjoys being treated like she is cheap and sleazy.

It's not just the guys; it's also the girls. They can get very bitchy with me and I've lost a few friends since becoming a model. One girl, who I will call Sandra (not her real name) who I'd been friends with since I was young, began to spread really malicious rumours about me, just because I was getting work and she wasn't.

I hardly go out clubbing any more and, if I do, it's with my boyfriend. I tend to cover up a lot more now because of the way people treat me. Maybe it will get better when I have my breast reduction.

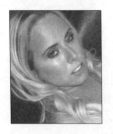

SARAH LOU

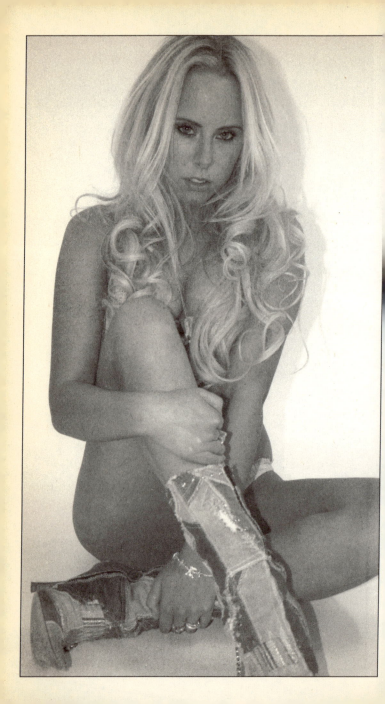

SARAH LOU

Name: Sarah Tottle
Model/Dance Name: Sarah Lou
Star Sign: Libra
Age: 20
Vital Stats: 32C-22-32
Lives: County Durham
Fave Food: Indian
Fave Drink: JD and Diet Coke

Where do you work?
Although I live in Durham, I normally work in London. A recent shoot I did in London was for tabloid girls' website, www.tabloidgirls.com. It's a website all about Page 3 girls and models that are in the tabloids. I also do other work such as the Maxpower Live shows, which are really exciting, because there are lots of other girls there and the atmosphere is buzzing.

I've not done a great deal of work outside the UK, but I did manage to get to Malta for a beauty shoot.

How did you get into modelling?

I was entered into a modelling contest when I was 18. I came second. It gave me a lot of confidence and so I started to enter more competitions. The more successful I became, the more I thought about doing this for a career. The next step was to join a few modelling agencies and the work started from them.

To date I have appeared in a two-page spread in *Redline*, Page 3 of the *Sport*, centre pages of the *Daily Star* Miss Cleavage. I have also been in magazines such as *Fast Car* and *Zoo* etc. I have been in the *People* newspaper, but that was for a sex story I sold about me and Gus out of *EastEnders*.

Getting into the modelling world was really difficult at first, as I live in Durham and all the work is in London. But I was ambitious and had lots of drive, so I never gave up. I just kept pushing myself. A lot of the work I get myself is through word of mouth. I also have a good friend, who I met through a photo shoot, who runs an agency and she has helped me a lot.

SARAH LOU

What's the biggest fee/tip you have ever earned?
The biggest fee I have earned to date is £4,000 – it was for the sex story I sold to the *Sunday People* and *Sunday Sport* about me and Gus from *Easties*.

Which highstreet publications have you been in? Have you worked with any famous people?
I have been in lots of print media, such as the *People*, the *Sun*, the *Daily Star*, the *Daily Sport*, *Closer* magazine, *Redline*, *Fast Car*, *Maxim*, *Max Power*, *Performance Bike*. I have also appeared in Channel 4's *Sex, Footballers and Videotapes* as well as Sky One's *Dream Team*.

I've met lots of famous people at model parties, such as *Playboy* party, *Loaded*, Supermodels UK, *ICE* mag's party etc. You can always expect to meet lots of celebrities at these kind of parties, such as Gary Lucy, Jordan, Jennifer Ellison, Jodie Marsh, Dev from *Corrie*, Ryan Giggs, Mohammed George, Dwight Yorke, Jeff Brazier etc.

What other work have you done?
I'm a full-time model now. But I have a good education to fall back on. I was always very athletic when I was younger and attended a dance school at Gateshead College, where I gained a BTEC in dance. I also competed for seven years as

TELL ME A SECRET

a gymnast – I can still do the splits! I did manage to get three AS levels, an A level and a Sports Coaching Award, CSLA.

I left Roseberry Sport and Community College (formally known as Roseberry Comp), with 2A*, 7As, 2Bs and 1C. Because of such outstanding results I was awarded the Bainbridge Trophy.

When I finished education I began working as a full-time receptionist at a garage and entered modelling competitions in my spare time. I was a finalist in the *Sun* Page 3 idol, came second in a *Daily Sport* competition, second in the *Max Power* Live Final 10. After only a few months of doing this I gave up my job at the garage and became a full-time model.

I think that once my modelling has finished I'd really like to get into TV presenting or acting, but not in the area of criminology or journalism.

Do you have any famous friends?

I wouldn't really call them friends, they are not like the ones I have at home. I have hung out with a few of them, such as Mohammed George, who plays Gus in *EastEnders*. I remember when Mohammed and me watched *Scary Movie 2* together. I have also shared a bed with Gary Lucy from *Footballers' Wives* series (read more later!). I was also out with Jodie Marsh at the Embassy and we were flashing at everyone – never a dull moment when you hang out with these people!

What does your family think of the work you do?

My family are really supportive. My dad was a bit wary at first. I remember one time when I first got into modelling, I was doing a shoot in Magaluf and he rang me to see if I was posing nicely – bless. It was a bit of a shock when my dad first saw me topless. My sister really loves what I do and would love to do the same.

I think my family are really happy for me, because I had it a bit rough whilst I was growing up. I was bullied while at school. It all started from a comment some lads from the 6th form said. They said that they thought I was the best-looking girl there and this really pissed off one particular girl. She started bullying me emotionally. She did a good job; within no time I was an outcast. I became depressed. This led to an eating disorder and I was in hospital for over a year.

I got my revenge on her in the end. I started dating the guy she adored. We are still together now and very happy and just about to move into our second home.

These people that treated me like an outcast, now come up to me in clubs and tell me how brilliant I am. I just rub it in their faces to get back at them. I still get a few girls saying I'm doing porn (something I would never consider doing – ever). I know they are just jealous and want me to look bad … get a life, girls.

What's your funniest moment?
I can't really think of one particular moment – there are so many. When you mix in the circles I do, it's a laugh a minute.

What's your scariest moment?
It was just after I started modelling and I was at a shoot in London with Jeff Kaine. I didn't have enough money for a hotel and had spent what little I had getting around London and buying a bit of lunch.

When I got to the train station I discovered that I had missed all the trains back home that evening and there was no other way to get back home. I decided that I would wait overnight at Victoria Station until I could get my train. I was really scared; there were a lot of dodgy characters hanging around, but I didn't have any choice.

It felt like an eternity sat in the station; I kept my head down, avoiding eye contact with anyone so as not to engage in conversation with the swarm of nutters that was gradually making their way into the station.

I'm not sure what would have happened to me if it hadn't been for my 'knight in shining armour'. A local cabby approached me and asked if I was OK. I must have looked like a little lost girl. He was real friendly, and I don't know why, maybe because I was so relieved to hear a friendly voice, but I started to cry. I started to explain what had happened and how scared I was. He took me to his car where it was lovely and warm and drove me around London. He bought a hot drink and some chips for me, then dropped me back at Victoria Station when my train was due. Thank you, Mr Cabby.

Have you ever turned down work and why?
I have turned down every job that's not nicely done or is pornographic. I would never pose nude or in top-shelf mag material. I think that kind of work isn't nice and it's degrading.

I don't like working with amateurs, because I just get the idea that they aren't really after the pics for anything else but their own 'personal' use – if you know what I mean? I get emails all the time asking me to pose for them. I generally ignore them.

TELL ME A SECRET

Do you have a sexual fantasy?
I would love a threesome with my fiancé and Colin Farrell. Not sure my fiancé would approve, but, hey, it's only a fantasy.

What's your most memorable sexual experience?
My boyfriend and me were still living with our parents so we had sex in all kinds of places. I remember one time we had gone to a house party. We had drunk loads and were pretty wasted, but very horny. We decided that it would be OK to have sex in the field behind the house where the party had been. What we hadn't banked on was that people use the field to cut across. We were well at it when we spotted a couple cutting across the field. We stopped as they passed, but we were having too much of a good time to stop completely, so we carried on until we had both come.

What do you think about group sex? Have you tried it?
I won't try it and never have. I think sex should be with someone you love and respect. I don't judge people who do it, it's up to them. Most couples do it to spice up their own sex lives, but there are better things to do – just visit an Ann Summers shop!!

SARAH LOU

What advice would you give someone who wanted to get into this business?
Don't fall into the traps that are out there and join reputable agencies. It's a good lifestyle and you can get respect as long as you don't get exploited and join a bad agency.

Which bloke do you fancy the most?
Colin Farrell.

Tell me a secret ... I'm not sure why I haven't told anyone about this. It's not like it's a shameful secret or anything. It was more a bit of fun. I think it was because some people would think it was odd and not see the funny side of it.

It all started when I was at a *Playboy* party, hosted by Natalie Denning. While I was there I met Gary Lucy from *Footballers' Wives*. My friend, Emily, that I had met at the party and me went back to Gary's place in Essex for more drinks. I was pretty pissed and was at the stage where I just needed to sleep, so I staggered upstairs and found a bed to crash in.

When I woke up, I discovered that it was Gary's bed and he was next to me. However, I don't think he noticed that I had woken up, as he was shagging the hell out of my friend, Emily, who was also in the same bed. It was really embarrassing.

TELL ME A SECRET

A few weeks later I was back in London and needed somewhere to stay. I knew my new friend, Emily, lived close to London, in Cambridge. Even though I'd only ever met her once at the *Playboy* party, when we went back to Gary Lucy's house, she was a good laugh and I knew she wouldn't mind me staying at hers, so I gave her a call.

I had finished my casting, but Emily was still on a shoot when I called. So I got the cab straight to the shoot. The shoot had over-run and she was running late. I had to be in another part of London for my next shoot, so we arranged to meet up later on in the day.

I headed to King's Cross station, where we had arranged to meet, in order to get the train to Cambridge. However, she turned up with the male model she had been working with on the shoot. She was all over him. He suggested that we all get a hotel and not head back to Cambridge.

We found a hotel and he ordered a triple room for us. They had an alcoholic drink and I had a cappuccino. I sensed the chemistry between them straight away. I went to bed and they were at it almost straight away in the bed next to me. I tried to get to sleep, but they were f***ing for hours.

I lay there wondering whether every time I went out with Emily I would be voyeur to her sexual activities. It just seemed really funny that both times I had been out with Em I had watched her perform!

The guy left the next morning and kept ringing Em up, but she didn't want anything to do with him. He had a girlfriend anyway. We had some filming to do for *Sex, Footballers and Videotapes* on Channel 4 at Tantra Nightclub that night and he rang her non-stop.

I went home up north afterwards and I rang Emily a week later and she told me that she had got together with him. Then I spoke to her again and she was still with him and he had met 'the parents'.

However, a few weeks after that a story in the newspaper had said Emily was dating Lee from Blue. You have to give it to her; she definitely knows how to enjoy herself.

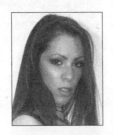

NADINE PELE

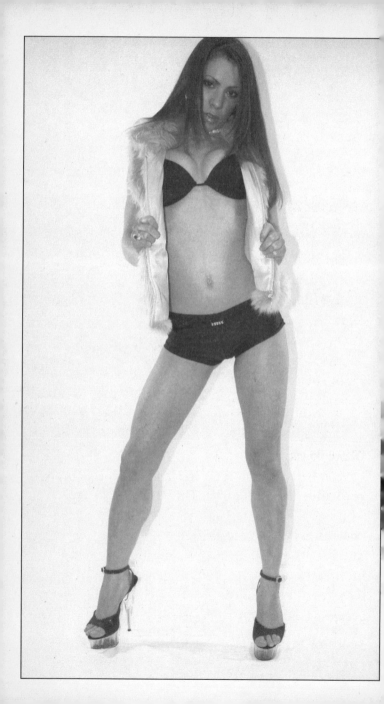

NADINE PELE

Name: Nadine Pele
Model/Dance Name: Nadine Pele
Star Sign: Capricorn
Age: 22
Vital Stats: 32B-24-32
Lives: Norwich
Fave Food: Pasta
Fave Drink: Cranberry and orange juice

Where do you work?
I live in Norwich but I'm a freelance model, so my work takes me around the UK.

How did you get into modelling?
My dad always wanted me to be a model. I think I must have been the pretty little girl who could turn heads. Even his friends used to bring me presents when I was younger, they thought I was so cute.

My first modelling job was for Grattons catalogue. I think the shoot was in London, but I was only eight and was so excited, so for all I know it could have been in Timbuktu. My dad's friend had two daughters aged ten and six, who were with us. We all looked the same (pretty with long dark hair). All I can really remember is being in a studio and having to keep changing the clothes. I can never remember ever seeing the pictures in a catalogue so it could have been my first-ever test shoot. Even then I was showing off and loving the camera.

The glamour photography was just something that happened – JC (my photographer) organised a fashion shoot for his own portfolio. There were meant to be five other models turning up. One of the male models knew me and it was from his recommendation that I was there.

JC went wild when he saw me; he thought I was great and we quickly arranged a shoot where it would be just me. The other models (who were meant to be professionals) were really wooden. At the end of the shoot he paid me (I was not there to be paid as far as I was concerned it was just to get a few pics for my portfolio). The next shoot he suggested the clothed glamour shots. I enjoyed it and the images he provided for me were great.

NADINE PELE

I could never imagine doing a boring 9–5 job forever. I'm too hyperactive and always have been. I went to Earlham High School, Norwich and my favourite lesson was Sports (PE). I had a teacher called Miss Levey who was concerned that I took speed – apparently I was very hyper and energetic while at school. Like all good schoolgirls, I also had an active imagination, so I inevitably had a crush on a teacher, Mr Siviter. He was head of my year and was a dish! I used to get into trouble so I could be in detention with him – if he only knew (oops, maybe he does now). I also had a bit of a crush on Mr Ranger who was the Deputy Head; he was ever so nice and lovely and he really did care about the pupils.

What's the biggest fee/tip you have ever earned?

Biggest tip – I gave £3 to a taxi driver. Oh, you mean for me? The biggest fee to date is the first ever glamour shoot with JC. He paid me £100 for two hours' work – he has also given me a website, prints and a load of advice and direction, so you could say I got a bonus!

The shoot only took place in a small studio in Norwich, but it was great (who said size matters!). I love working with JC as he gets the best out of me. Even my friends who have met him love him.

TELL ME A SECRET

What other work have you done?

I am at Norwich City College on Ipswich Road studying Spanish (Preliminary Level). I love studying, although I feel really out of place in the class as they are all dead posh and there's scruffy old me with a Norfolk accent – I suppose I will be the only one who can speak Spanish and sound like I come from a farm in Spain.

Before that, I went to college to study for a make-up artist diploma. I knew that I was good. I would make my friends up before we went to college and even now, at the age of 22, I am still putting it on for them.

Unfortunately, I had to quit my course early, because the place where I lived could not handle my dog (I have a lovely big Dobermann bitch) and I ended up in a shared house (which is a book in itself).

Apart from my modelling I have always wanted to work as cabin crew. When I was 12, I wrote to Richard Branson (with help from my dad) with dreams of becoming one of his 'faithful airhostesses'. I think his reply said for me to write back when I was 18, which I never did, as he has a height restriction of 5'6". I can remember hearing about the height restriction and I cried for hours because I always wanted to work for him. My dad cuddled and reassured me that there were other airlines I could work for. I didn't tell him, as I didn't want him to feel helpless, but I was secretly shattered. I only ever wanted to work for Virgin.

I could do any job really, as long as it revolved around me being centre of attention – acting, model or a dancer. My dream job would be to model for Versace (one can hope). I would really like to work as a children's TV presenter, although the kids might just be a little taller than me.

I wouldn't say no to a job as the personal trainer for Brian Harvey. When I was about 12, I loved East 17. My friend Kerry saw this article about him saying that Mariah Carey would be his ideal bird. At the time everyone said that I was a spit of her so I was smitten – I wonder if he is free now?

Unlike most glamour models, I refuse to ever be in the class of a Page 3 or a *Sunday Sport* model. My dad always told me that I am 'class not brass'. Glamour is not always about cheesy tit shots that end up being next day's fish and chip wrapping!

Do you have any famous friends?

I don't have any famous friends, but am lucky to have some loyal close friends, who may one day be famous – ask me again in another five years!

TELL ME A SECRET

What does your family think of the work you do?
Before my dad died, it was his wish for me to be a model. He died early in 2004. Thankfully it was while he was asleep so it would not have been painful. I do miss him; he was the keystone in my life. Everything I did was for him and he supported everything that I did. I know all daughters will say this, but no one could love their dad as much as I loved mine.

All of my family who have seen my pictures think it's great and none of them treats me as an air-head. They know I am focused and I will achieve my aims.

What's your funniest moment?
It was on a trip to Blackpool. I went with a couple of friends and, basically, I was pissed the whole weekend. It was wicked. I remember going to Funny Girls, a bar full of drag queens, some were really pretty and some looked like Lily Savage. The shows that they did were really good and the dresses they wore were amazing. Every single drag queen looked like they were seven foot tall and the bodies were better than a lot of real girls could ever wish for.

All I can remember on the Saturday is that we started drinking in the afternoon and then hitting the Pleasure Beach. I bought this huge burger and followed it off with popcorn and candy floss. It was just a bad combination with all the rides. I felt sick before I even went on the ride. Rather worse for wear, I boarded the Grand National – it's a race between two roller coasters. Anyway, by the time the ride got to the top of the first hill, I was really suffering and possibly the height did it for me. I threw up all over the backs of the riders in front – I cannot repeat what they said but it wasn't pleasant – to be honest, I couldn't care less at this point. I was just glad that I had thrown up, because it made me feel a lot better. My mates were really embarrassed about the whole thing and really gave me loads of grief about it. I have never drunk that much since and certainly won't mix Jack Daniels with Malibu ever again.

Another funny time was when I was about 15 and I was at a friend's house and getting drunk playing spin the bottle (yes, I was only 15). One guy at the party got really drunk. I didn't like him; he was being loud and showing off. Finally, he passed out on the couch. Me, being the bitch, decided to pour water over the crotch area of his jeans. He was asleep for a little while longer and the rest of us were playing a computer game. All I remember was as soon as he woke up he rushed out of the room and out of the house.

Nobody ever mentioned it to him, so he actually thought he had pissed himself. It was only when I started dating him 18 months later that I told him that it was me – he went berserk – but he loved me and forgave me. I knew then that I had a knack for getting men to love me no matter what I did to them – just ask all of my exes.

What's your scariest moment?

A few of us had gone round a friend's house in Norwich. I was 12 at the time. It was nearly 11pm so my friend and I decided to make our way home. The road was fairly busy even though it was late. Suddenly a car stopped and this guy got out and walked over to us. He asked us loads of questions and asked if we took cocaine or other drugs. He grabbed our arms when we tried to walk off and tried to get us in his car. We both were quite streetwise for our age and we both laid into him. He released us and we ran off. The worst thing was that two police cars passed us (don't forget we are only 12), even though we tried to flag them down and they still didn't stop – it was only when we pretended to have a fight that the next police car stopped.

I know that it was a horrible thing to think but at the time I was glad it happened because I knew

I was in for a tremendous bollocking for being out so late.

The guy ended up going to jail – I hated going to court and was very nervous. Leading up to the trial we only had a few interviews, which were scary in themselves, but it was my dad who was there for me. His strength was huge, he was a man of very strong moral principles, which I think if he hadn't been he would probably have killed the guy. I suspect that the thought was there.

The guy was sent down for a year. I do see him occasionally in Norwich (the last time in the main mall only a couple of weeks ago) and he does look at me but I'm not sure if he recognises me or not. He would have to be very stupid to try it with me now; I am fairly strong and not a little 12-year-old any more.

Have you ever turned down work and why?

JC advises me on the modelling jobs and the filming tests. He has a knack of weeding out the prats, perverts and time wasters. He will make me ask pertinent questions. For instance I was going to go to Hertfordshire for a test for a movie. The guy said it could be only be done on a Monday or Tuesday. JC volunteered to take me, but I would have to arrange it for the weekend as that was the only time he could take me. The guy refused and said it had to be Monday or Tuesday – then he said the test would have to be at his house. JC got me to phone him and ask, if it was at his house, why couldn't it be at the weekend. The next question was, had a producer viewed the script – the guy admitted that the script was still being written – I basically told him to get back to me when he was seriously ready for casting sessions.

I do get emails from dirty old men that want to shoot me in lingerie. To be honest, even though it means I am losing out on money, I really do not want to see bad images of me. If I am ever lucky enough to be famous, then those kinds of images will return to haunt me.

Do you have a sexual fantasy?
I don't really have any at the moment.

What's your most memorable sexual encounter?
My most memorable encounter of sex is when I was caught with a boyfriend (no names) in a cemetery. It was during the day and three oldies that were visiting caught us. The thing is getting caught was the best bit about it as the rest was too bloody uncomfortable and cold to really rank in the best sessions I have ever had.

NADINE PELE

What do you think about group sex? Have you ever tried it?
Group sex – not my bag but each to their own. So, no.

What advice would you give to someone who wanted to get into this business?
My advice for someone starting out is to find a friend who will help you. Stand back and listen to other people's advice and then give an opinion.

Maybe hook up with an amateur photographer, they need the practice as much as you do. It has worked great for me. I have got a lot more confident and Steve, the guy who has done all of my photography, has also benefited greatly.

Which bloke do you fancy the most?
Russell Crowe (especially when looking rough).

Tell me a secret ... It started with an argument with my mum when I was still at school – I was a terrible teenager and a right bitch: paranoid of everything about myself, so highly strung to every comment. I cannot remember what the argument was about – probably something very lame, but I ran out and promised never to come back.

I knew a girl who had her own council flat and

she always left her key in a secret hiding place (I knew where, of course). I moped around her house. After a few hours I heard her voice, I could also hear a man's voice and they were coming up the drive. I panicked and quickly hid under her bed – I don't know why really, as she wouldn't have minded me being there.

I won't mention her name, but if she gets to read this she will know who she is. What happened next shocked the hell out of me. Not long after she got in, it was fairly obvious that she was having sex in the front room. What was more shocking was when she came into the bedroom; I could see three pairs of feet. It really freaked me out. I could not believe it of my friend, as I always thought she was great. I felt she had betrayed me by being so dirty.

The sex she had was very aggressive. You have to remember I was a 15 year-old virgin and basically experiencing my first sexual encounter from under a bed. It was disgusting; they were f***ing her hard and she was loving it. I could hear lots of moans and groans and slopping. They were saying things like, 'You love it, don't you, dirty f***ing bitch!'

Then the strangest thing happened, the moans were getting louder and more frantic, when suddenly she started making a braying sound just like a donkey when she had an orgasm. The guys laughed and sounded like they were trying to gag her. It was so degrading.

I would say they were at it for about an hour before the two men left. All the time I was laid as flat as possible and had my hands over my mouth trying not to make a single noise when I took a breath.

After the men had left, she went to get a shower and that's when I sneaked out. I really did lose all respect for her. I had always thought of her as my role model and after that 'sex fest' I could only see her as a slag. I knew she wasn't seeing anyone at the time and you could tell by the conversation that she had only just met these two men. They must have thought their luck had really come in that day. She was very pretty and had an awesome body – what a 'spitroasting' event! If she reads this, she will know why I stopped hanging around and maybe a few others will guess who the slag is.

I never told her that I was there. I did tell my mum though. I got home at about 1am. My mum was beside herself with worry and my dad just stayed out of the way. I ended up telling my mum about what happened and I think she soon realised how much the whole episode disturbed me. We still had arguments but I never ran away from home as it's the worst thing in the world to see your mother in tears because of you.

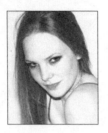

KERRI D

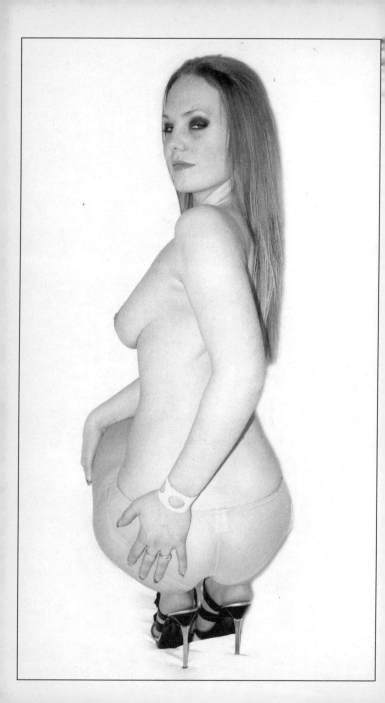

KERRI D

Name: Kerrie Davies
Model Name: Kerri D
Star Sign: Gemini
Age: 20
Vital Stats: 34D-24-34
Lives: Hastings
Fave Food: Indian
Fave Drink: Sex on the Beach

Where do you work?
I am based in Hastings but work all over Europe.

How did you get into modelling?
I started modelling from the age of about three – at Debenham's toddler competitions to local fashion shows. I first started glamour modelling when I was about 16, after several years of realising I wasn't getting any taller. I knew I

would never make it as a fashion model and this was the next best thing.

So one day I just took the plunge and thought, F*** it and booked a test shoot. I was slightly apprehensive about this career path, but very quickly I realised I was actually enjoying the work. I've stuck with it every since and I'm now at the point where I love what I do and wouldn't want to do anything else.

When I think about being a glamour model, the more I think that it is the perfect job for me. I have always wanted to be centre of attention – and, let me tell you, I get plenty of attention when I get my tits out!

What's the biggest fee/tip you have ever earned?
I'm just about to sign a £30K deal – that will definitely be my biggest to date.

What highstreet publications have you been in?
I have only just recently started to get somewhere with my modelling but so far I have been in *Loaded* magazine, *FHM*, *Nuts* magazine, *Max Power* magazine, *Max Power* Live show in Birmingham and have just been asked to be in *Fast Car* – and, obviously, not forgetting this book.

KERRI D

What other work have you done?

I usually end up working in London, as most of the work is there. I do occasionally manage to get local jobs, which is great when you land a job on your doorstep. Most of my modelling work has been for magazines and websites, mainly promotional work. I get a lot of regular work via websites such as www.toplessbabe.co.uk, www.toplessbabez.com & www.kerridavies.co.uk, which is my own site.

The best job has got to be when I did *Loaded* magazine, not particularly for the assignment, but for the buzz that I got from it. It was almost like my first wake-up call to what my life could be like if I pushed myself. It was great the way I was treated, the make-up artists, hair stylists, outfit designer – it was brilliant and I loved every minute of it.

I know at the end of the day I won't be looking like this forever, unless I meet a good plastic surgeon, so I am quite happy to be doing other things if it all falls through. My main priority is the man in my life, my son Ryan-Daniel who is nearly four. He's the funniest thing in the world and the best thing that's ever happened to me. I'm pretty level-headed when it comes to a modelling career. It can be a nightmare worrying about my son and making sure he is being looked after when I'm working. I have turned down lots of jobs due to things like not being able to pick my son up from nursery on time etc. But no matter whether it was *Playboy* or an assignment in the tropics, if my son were ill, I'd be right back with my baby, without a doubt.

Just in case my modelling career doesn't give me a decent living, I'm also currently at college studying IT, which makes everyone laugh considering I'm meant to be a 'dumb blonde glamour model'.

Do you have any famous friends?
I have 'contacts' as I like to call it – ha ha.

My cousin is Shwan Jalal, who plays for Tottenham, so I tend to know more footballers than anyone else. I have met quite a few famous people, but I still prefer to be friends with my 'normal' friends that were there before I became a model and will be there long after it ends.

I had a phone call recently from my cousin, Shwan, he was laughing down the phone saying he had just seen me in *Nuts* magazine. He said that he had some lads that wanted to talk to me. I was driving through Hastings town centre, so I couldn't exactly have a conversation and then all I heard was loads of blokes shouting and hollering. I just thought it was my cousin's mates taking the piss, so I hung up.

KERRI D

Not long after, I was speaking to Shwan and he asked why I hung up the phone when his mates wanted to speak to me. I just told him that I thought that they were taking the piss. He laughed and explained that he was just about to go on to the pitch when he saw all the boys from Woking football team round a magazine. My cousin went over and, to his embarrassment, it was his little cousin they were all looking at. They didn't believe it when Shwan said I was his cousin and that's when he called me. How embarrassing? But I have to admit I got a good buzz from it.

Celebrities always meant a lot to me when I was growing up – what they looked like, or what they wore. So when Shwan got signed up to Tottenham I thought it was amazing that one of my family was going to be famous. Slowly he started getting places with his football; it was unreal the way he would talk about things and names such as Stephen Gerrard and Teddy Sherringham just popped up as though it was the norm. I was totally star-struck by the thought of these people. It was wicked.

What does your family think of the work you do?

My mum was OK, in fact, shockingly OK. She came with me to my first shoot, which I wasn't too keen on at first. I wasn't sure if she was being supportive, or whether it was a clever way to get me to back down. She very bluntly said to me, 'Kerri, if you want to do it, just do it, I will support you no matter what', which couldn't have been more perfect.

But my dad, well, there is a different story all together. He didn't quite see it the way my mum did. He didn't like the thought of his little girl taking her clothes off for money, which I guess is most fathers' reaction.

I will never forget how my dad dealt with it. He thought that, if he ignored it, it might just go away. But the more he ignored it, the more magazines I started to appear in. Then one day I finally plucked up the courage to show him.

I was visiting my nan, showing her the *Loaded* magazine that I had just appeared in. Nan was great, she just smiled and sniggered, saying, 'Oh dear, what are you like.' While I was showing my nan, my dad walked in. At first I thought, Oh bugger, but figured, if I didn't show him now, someone else would. I took a deep breath and said, 'Dad, what do you think of this?' Then proudly opened up the mag right in his face. He just stared to start off with. My heart was racing, wondering how he was going to react. Finally, he said, 'Oh, that's OK, innit?' I laughed, partly with relief and partly 'cause I saw a slight glimmer of proudness in there somewhere. His reaction brought a tear to my eye, it made me happier than he will ever know – obviously he will now when he reads this – whoops!

I hope when this book is published he might start to realise how well I'm doing in my modelling career and be proud of me. However, since the episode at my nan's, he's actually started asking about jobs, rather than criticising them.

But back to my mum, she has always been so cool, it's brilliant. Like one time, she rang me from the supermarket to ask what magazine I was in. She was shouting down the phone, 'Kerrie, I'm in Safeways, what magazine are you in?' I could hear her fumbling through the mags. She managed to find it while being on the phone to me. Still chatting away, she got to the check-out desk and I could hear her saying to the check-out person, 'Oh yeah, you see her, that's my daughter, isn't she lovely?' Oh my God, I just wanted to die, how embarrassing. I started shouting, 'Mum! Shut up! What are you like?' She is very funny, bless her.

My brother, Daniel, died in August 1997 – I would have loved to have had his approval. But somehow I know that he approves and is watching me make something of myself.

TELL ME A SECRET

What's your funniest moment?

All in all I guess I have got to say some of my funniest moments are when I'm out with friends in my local town, Hastings, on a piss-up.

I always have a good laugh with them. One time and I know she is going to hate me for it – sorry Jo – a load of us were all out in Hastings, drinking in our usual haunts like Yates, Weatherspoons, French's, before hitting Waves nightclub in George Street, Hastings. We were all dancing, making idiots of ourselves. I turned round to see my mate Jo, who had been heading back from the bar, slip over. But, as she did, she was mid-falling over and controlling it (in a pissed kinda way!) and was sliding around steadying herself getting back on her feet. It was comical, as she must have been sliding around for about four minutes, slight exaggeration, but it did feel like a long time. I kept thinking, Why doesn't she just fall and get it over with? I was crying with laughter, but I still went to try and help her. As I approached her, I skidded on the wet floor, kicked her over and we both fell on our arses. We lay there for minutes laughing too much to get up. I nearly pissed myself and daren't get up in case gravity got the better of my bladder. Luckily we were pretty hammered so the huge bruises, which we discovered the next day, didn't hurt. Typical Saturday night really!

KERRI D

I have fun whoever I'm with and wherever I am, even when I'm working. For instance I had a modelling assignment in Spain in March 2004; I went with another model Kiki – aka Tasha. We had such a giggle. We were meant to be on location the whole time we were there, but it didn't turn out that way as we got in trouble everywhere we went. We were nearly thrown out of a Chinese restaurant for a slight accident when a pearl necklace broke and went all over the floor. Everyone in the restaurant was on their hands and knees trying to pick up the pieces, and people were nearly falling over – it was hysterical and just a little bit embarrassing.

What's your scariest moment?

When I first started modelling I got myself an agent. One day my agent gave me a contact number, saying this bloke wants to do a shoot with me and that I had to ring him to set it up. Still a bit naïve as to how things work, I agreed. I should have thought, Hang on, isn't that my agent's job? Well, like everything, you learn from your mistakes.

Anyway, I rang this man and he seemed OK, asking me what kind of work I did and what I wanted to do. I felt happy with the situation, so we made the arrangements for the shoot.

It got to the day of the shoot and still my agent hadn't called to let me know the details of the assignment and where he wanted to meet before the shoot. So I rang him and he said, 'Oh no, darling, you'll be fine going on your own. He's OK, he is a nice bloke.' I immediately felt uncomfortable and it didn't feel right going on my own, so I called my friend and asked her to come with me.

I was all set, but last minute I thought I should call the photographer and inform him that I would be with a friend, as some photographers don't like spectators. Oh my God, did this 'nice bloke' turn psycho on me. Within a second he started being really funny with me, saying that I had to come on my own or the shoot would be cancelled. It freaked me out, and there was no way I was going to be with this nutter on my own, so I told him to stick it.

A short while later, he must have got my email address off my agent. I started to get these emails asking to re-schedule to another time. He was mentioning hotels and saying that he wanted to choose the outfit, as he knew what he wanted to see me in that would do it for him. I was completely freaked out by this weirdo; he kept changing from nice one minute to a psycho the next. It was horrible, almost like he had turned into a stalker or something. After a few visits to the police station, luckily I didn't hear any more. But that didn't put me off modelling, just made me wiser. I got myself another agent and am just about to sign a £30K deal so glad I kept with it.

Have you ever turned down work and why?
Yes, I have turned down quite a few jobs because of the inconvenience, owing to being a mum. For example, flying off to Portugal at a day's notice – a bit hard to sort childcare out in 12 hours.

The most annoying jobs that I turn down every single day of my life are the offers of porn. I haven't got anything against it, but it's just not my cuppa tea – plus my mum would kill me. Lap dancing/pole dancing is my next aim. I love it; the girls look so sexy and powerful and in control, with men just completely dazzled. It's brilliant.

I am constantly being asked to do porn, or to do Girl/Girl stills and things like that and, trust me, it's a very easy way of making money. There are always sleazy guys that you get email job offers from, they all want open-leg shots or want you to do a private show and dress up like a schoolgirl or something – they are sick and need help.

Do you have a sexual fantasy?
My sexual fantasy, mmmm, picture this – a

waterfall in the mists of a tropical forest, the hot sun beating down. My boyfriend and I are swimming in the secluded waters to cool down. We start to kiss, his hands running over my body. As we make our way under the waterfall he takes off my bikini, his hands and mouth caressing every inch of my body. As the cold icy waters pounds down on us, I wrap my legs around his waist pushing myself down on him, feeling him deep inside. Our bodies move in perfect time, kissing more and more passionately, holding each other so tight. Then with one last grind of our bodies we both have an unbelievable wild climax. Guess where I'm going on my holiday? Yes, somewhere hot, with a waterfall!

What's your most memorable sexual encounter?
I don't think you can really say which is your best sexual encounter. I think it's just a certain time that you just think, Oh my God, that was amazing, and, luckily and thankfully, I can say that often with my man. Me and my fella have the best sex ever, definitely 10 out of 10 in the bedroom.

What do you think about group sex? Have you tried it?
Group sex isn't something I think, Yuk! That's disgusting, because I don't think it is disgusting. I

think, if you are in the situation where you have the opportunity to do it and you're not hurting anyone and no one is attached or anything, then I think it's cool. I'd do it if it meant everyone was happy and no one was getting hurt, why not? I think it would definitely be an experience you wouldn't forget in a hurry.

I have been asked to do a threesome quite a few times, but never taken them up on the offer. I think if the person I loved wanted to have a threesome, then I would. I'm not being pervy or anything, but, if it's something that he had thought about and wanted to do, I'd rather him do it with me than with someone else. However, there are conditions – the third person would have to be one of two things: a complete stranger that we had never seen before, or someone really close to us so that we knew where they had been and felt comfortable with them. But then on the other hand if my bloke ever asked me to have a threesome I'd probably be too shocked, panic, smack him in the mouth and dump him – ha ha.

What advice would you give to someone who wanted to get into this business?

This business is definitely one to go into with your eyes open. Apart from the perverts that are out there flashing their cash in temptation, it's a really tough competitive career. The whole time you are on an emotional roller coaster, one minute getting great jobs, the next being told you are not good enough. For every job you land, you are rejected for 10. Until you are in this industry you don't realise how many girls in the world are trying to make it – there's millions. And yet the only household names you hear are Katie Price, aka Jordon, Jakki Degg, Caprice etc.

I think if I had to give advice to someone who wanted to get into the industry it would be: be prepared for the knock-backs, get a good portfolio together, enter competitions and promote yourself as much as you can. I promote myself mainly through the web and get a lot of work from them. I advertise on anything and everything from websites, other agencies, even down to modelling pictures with my website printed on the thong!

If you're not going to put in more than 110%, then question yourself, is it really for you? I want to know that, in 10 years' time if no one knows my name, at least I can say I tried and have had no regrets and that I couldn't have done anything differently.

Which bloke do you fancy the most?
Vin Diesel.

KERRI D

Tell me a secret ... A short while ago I was having a really shit time, my life was crap and I was having it real rough. It all started when my boyfriend had gone on holiday to the Dominican Republic for a two-week holiday with a group of friends. We had been together for a while and were hopelessly in love with each other. I felt miserable without him.

I had recently met up with a group of friends that I hadn't seen for a while. So, while my fella was away, rather than moping around the house, I spent all my time with these friends getting pissed, mostly. We were having a good laugh, going out enjoying ourselves and living life to the full. It really took my mind off missing my fella.

Everything was going OK, until someone, who I thought was a very close friend, decided to stab me in the back and started spreading rumours. One night we were having a drink and a laugh when I noticed one of my old friends looking really down and sad – he was going through a bit of a bad patch. Now anyone that knows me knows I am an easy person to talk to and always there to listen. I don't like to see people down, so I asked him if he was OK and said I was here if he needed a shoulder to cry on.

However, the narrow-minded people I was hanging around with saw only the worst in my friendship towards him. Rumours started, as they assumed that, because I was spending a lot of time with him, I was obviously f***ing him. I knew it was all bullshit, so I didn't think too much of it at first and either ignored their comments or laughed it off. I even mentioned it to my boyfriend when he called from his holiday. He just said, 'Well, you know how people like to gossip,' then he laughed and said, 'Just ignore them – I'm back soon and that will put a stop to their rumours.'

I continued going out with the same group of friends throughout the time my boyfriend was away because I didn't want to be on my own.

It was great when my bloke came home; I'd missed him like crazy. We couldn't keep our hands off each other; it felt like he had never been away. Then, not long after he got back, the rumours started getting worse. Again I didn't think too much of it, just wondered why people were so childish. I put it down to jealousy because of what I had with my boyfriend.

Then one day when I was just vegging around the house, my phone rang, and it was my boyfriend. He was screaming and shouting down the phone, 'You dirty f***ing bitch, you lied to me!' I was in shock, I tried to talk to him, but he wasn't listening. What the hell had I done? Had I missed something? He ordered me to get to his house immediately and hung up.

I was still trying to understand what I was meant to have done that was so bad that he would react like that. It was so out of character. My little boy was staying over at his gran's, so I quickly grabbed my jacket and headed off to his house. My heart was pounding the whole journey, and I was confused and upset all at the same time.

As I pulled up outside his house, he was outside waiting for me. He marched to my car and got into the passenger seat. He was shouting at me calling me all the names under the sun and more. 'You slept with that f***ing guy. I can't believe you shagged him, you dirty deceitful bitch.'

I just laughed. 'How pathetic, do me a favour,' I said. 'I wouldn't do that, you know I wouldn't.' My ex-boyfriend, who was my baby's father, had an affair and I know how much it hurt, so I wouldn't dream of doing that to anyone.

Nothing I said convinced him that I was innocent, so we went to the person in question's house to try and resolve the situation. Within two minutes of arriving at this guy's house, my boyfriend said to him, 'So tell me the truth, have you been sleeping with Kerrie?' There was this deadly silence for what seemed a lifetime, but must have only been seconds. Then this so-called friend, who I had put a lot of my time and effort in to trying to help, said, 'Yes, yes, I have.' At this point I went ballistic. I couldn't believe what he had said. I had helped this guy and he was causing me all this shit. Why? What reason did he have? What had I ever done to him, apart from show him friendship and kindness?

I screamed and shouted for my boyfriend to believe me. He just stood up, called me a whore and walked out of the house. I couldn't argue back, I was still in shock. I looked at the person I thought was my friend. He had a twisted look on his face, a look of self-triumph. What was this guy doing, did he realise the damage his lies were doing? Did he realise the hurt I was feeling?

In minutes I had lost the love of my life and someone who I thought was a friend. I was gutted. I felt sick to the stomach and my whole body trembled. I was sobbing when I ran out of the house and got into my car. My hands were shaking so much I could hardly start the car, then, with one almighty roar of the engine, I sped off. I didn't know where to go. I just drove erratically through the streets, nearly crashing two or three times. Then when I had run out of places to drive I knew I had to go home.

By the time I pulled up outside my house I was

crying so hysterically I couldn't see where I was going. The first thing I did when I got into the house was to grab the phone to try and call my boyfriend. I loved him so much and was not about to let go of him; I would do anything for him. When he did answer my calls he just shouted 'whore' and slammed the phone down on me.

If I were guilty then maybe it would have been easier to cope with. I would have deserved it. I understood his reaction; after all he thought I had cheated. I would have reacted in the same way if the roles had been reversed. But this twisted bastard had lied to split me and my boyfriend up, because secretly in his warped horrible mind he thought we would get together – yeah, right!

The more my boyfriend hung up on me the more hysterical I became. I was in a mess. That's when I did something stupid, something that I have not spoken about since, until now.

Sobbing hysterically I staggered into the kitchen. I couldn't see anything and was falling over things that were on the floor. I flung open the cupboard doors where I keep all my tablets and medicines and grabbed as many pills as I could and downed the lot.

To give you an idea of how many pills, there was nearly a full bottle of Paracetamol and about

45 Nighttime painkillers, normally you only need to take two to knock you out.

Still sobbing, I went back into the front room and tried to ring him again. He was not answering. 'Shit what have I done?' Suddenly I got a reality check. 'Oh my God, what have I done? My son needs me, what a selfish bitch!' I said this out loud over and over again. As I was saying this I started to feel light-headed. This is it, I thought, I'm going to die a sad, selfish bitch and leave my poor son motherless. All I could see was my son's beautiful face, his smile, I could smell him, feel him. With my son in mind, I got the strength to push myself in order to grab the phone and rang my mum. I don't know what I was saying, it was something like 'I've done something stupid', but by this time I was in and out of consciousness.

Next thing I remember was a paramedic standing over me, repeatedly saying my name. 'Kerrie, Kerrie, how many have you taken?' It all felt unreal. I don't know if I responded. I came to a few times in the ambulance on my way to the Conquest Hospital in Hastings.

The time in the hospital is still vague. I remember everyone being there, my mum, stepdad, dad, stepmum. I kept thinking I was tripping. I could see my boyfriend. He had come to the hospital but then the next time I opened my eyes he was gone. I remember at one point looking about and everyone was staring down at me – I couldn't speak, maybe I was dead. Everyone crying and upset. It was all my fault, how selfish was I?

I was finally discharged after having charcoal pumped into me, in order for me to vomit and lots of blood tests etc. I stayed with my mum for a few weeks. I just couldn't bring myself to go home and have all the memories of happier times with my boyfriend.

When I was strong enough I finally sent him a text message asking him if we could meet up to try and sort things out. He ignored the messages for a few days, but then agreed to meet. I didn't want to meet him to beg him to take me back; I just wanted him to believe me.

We did sort things out and are getting on with our lives – so a big 'F*** you' to all the people that tried ruining my life because it didn't work: we are in love and happy. As for my modelling career, well, just watch this space, I'm going to be a household name yet!

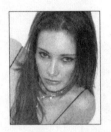

STACEY O'CONNELL

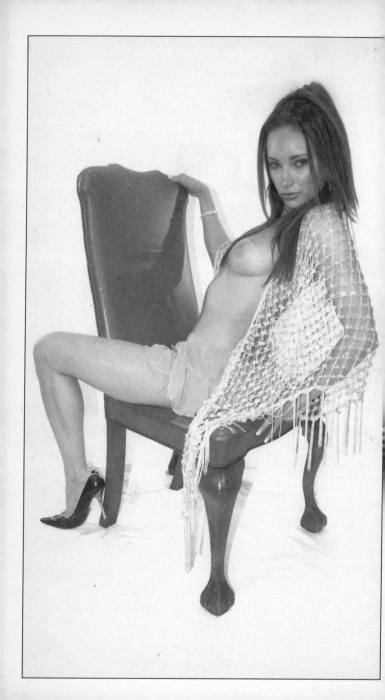

STACEY O'CONNELL

Name: Stacey O'Connell
Model/Dance Name: Stacey O'Connell
Star Sign: Aquarius
Age: 18
Vital Stats: 34C-26-34
Lives: Banstead, Surrey
Fave Food: Vindaloo curry
Fave Drink: Jack Daniels and Coke

Where do you work?

I'm currently a part-time model/part-time beautician and also do some legal contract work for friends in the modelling industry. I am self-employed with all of what I do.

The beautician work is with clients that I've kept since studying beauty at college. I travel to their homes and do my treatments there. The legal contract work is mainly done over the internet and my modelling work tends to be all based in the London area.

There are lots of studios around London. The work I did for the *Sun* was done in Alan Strutt's studio in London and the *Maxim* competition was done at Foxley Studios in Purley, Croydon.

I also occasionally travel and, in fact, I am due to travel to Dublin next week for shoots with two agencies I have out there. I have family over in Ireland, so it will be a bit of work and pleasure.

How did you get into modelling?

I was first spotted at the age 15. I was out with friends on Croydon High Street, when a talent scout approached me, asking if I'd ever considered modelling. I began my career with them and started out doing TV ads, catalogue and promotional work.

My next progression was when I was only 16 and that was to do my first fashion show for Rolanda Fashions at Hilton Hotel, London. It was with Zebramodels. The clothes were fabulous. All the other models were great with me and helped me along. It must have been obvious I was still a novice. When I saw the crowds I told them that I was paranoid that I would fall over! But they reassured me that even they, after years of experience, still have those thoughts going through their head.

I remember my first casting. I was very nervous, but dead excited at the same time. It was 'Dear Deirdre' for the *Sun* and I had to play a babysitter for a couple on New Year's Eve. After I had done this, I gained a lot of confidence and got on a lot better in the industry.

What's the biggest fee/tip you have ever earned?

I think my biggest fee to date was for a glamour photographer who made up a book of glamour images and used illusion photography. It was all very technical and clever. I ended up with £700 for a full day's modelling. Not a bad day's work.

What highstreet publications have you been in? Have you worked with any famous people?

My first taste of working with the top people was when I did the 'Dear Deirdre' with the *Sun*. This is where I developed most of my confidence in modelling and acting. Then I got my first fashion show when I joined Zebramodels at the age of 16. At this event I got to meet actors from *EastEnders*!

I succeeded in not falling over and was amazed at the adrenaline rush you get from being in front of so many cameras and famous people. After that I worked with many photographers for catalogues/club promotions/TV ads.

Then aged 18, my friend saw an advert in *The Stage* for Page 3 models for the *Sun* and asked me if I'd go along for moral support. We went there and surprisingly I was picked for a shoot with Alan Strutt, which I was shocked about, as I'd never even tried glamour modelling before. My friend didn't get in. She had fake breasts and the *Sun* wouldn't have her in the paper (which was very awkward for me at first, as I felt really bad for her). I decided, as I had been picked, that I might as well give it a go. I didn't expect to get anywhere, but was called back for another shoot a couple weeks later. At this point I was chuffed and happy to be working with Alan Strutt. Models like Zoë and Nicola are an inspiration for models like me.

I managed to come second in the Page 3 Idol competition 2004, which I can't exactly complain about as the girl that won was lovely and I got the exposure, which is good.

What other work have you done?

I have only done jobs that I am still doing. I still enjoy doing the beauty work and I think it helps with my career in modelling. It's a great skill to have in being able to do regular self-grooming. As

I'm qualified in manicures, pedicures, facials, waxing and facial bleaching etc, I save a fortune.

I get a lot of satisfaction doing my work. I love to make people look and feel their best. The legal work I do is mainly around drawing up legal contracts for models.

Apart from the above I am also a babysitter for my nephew, brothers and sisters. They are all under three! It can be a bit hectic in my house sometimes, especially with two dogs and two cats as well. Basically I live in a mad house!

Do you have any famous friends?

I think the most famous person I know would be the producer of Elite Models, Page 3 models, such as Nicola T and Zoë and the owner of Babe Station, Pat. That reminds me, I did some work at Babe Station when I'd just turned 18. I didn't want to do any more days! Fortunately, I worked there before it turned sleazy!

I also know Cal Packham, who works for national papers, and Alan Strutt from the *Sun*. I am in contact with Tess from *Maxim* mag and *Mayfair* magazine. I tried to persuade *Mayfair* magazine to let me do the mag with just a thong on! They wouldn't have though, so I declined the offer.

I wouldn't call any of them friends, more

contacts. Other than the above I don't know any more celebrities – YET.

What does your family think of the work you do?
My family was extremely happy when I first started out doing fashion work at 15/16. I think it was when I met Alan Strutt, Page 3, that it caused some conflict with my family.

When I first told my sister she was really happy for me and went around telling everyone at her college about it! My brother-in-law, who is Muslim, obviously had his own opinions on it, which was basically very clichéd and showed a big lack of understanding of what glamour modelling is. He saw it as if it was the same as selling myself! Which obviously shows the lack of knowledge about the modelling industry altogether. I gave as good as I got, so he now knows to keep his opinions to himself unless he wants a five-hour debate about it. We agree to disagree.

My dad had mixed feelings about it all. At first he couldn't understand why I'd do glamour, when I was doing OK with the commercial modelling. He didn't judge me though and he made sure I knew what I was getting into. He also made me aware of what other people's reactions would be, bearing in mind that my family are all Roman Catholic Irish. After a few months, he gradually told all his workmates and said he was proud of me. It took a while, but he got there in the end!

My mum also had mixed feelings, but came around after I promised her I wouldn't get into porn or anything like that!

My uncle John basically said well done and took the piss a bit but he was fine with it. He's not exactly Mr Perfect, so he knows how hard it is to succeed in life. My uncle Des was very proud and has since put some of my fashion pics up in his house, which is nice to know. As for my little bro, sis and nephew, I've got a good 10 years to think about how to tackle their reaction.

My nan was the biggest one to tell about it all, as she is very set in her ways about things and I knew her reaction wouldn't be good. I planned to tell her myself, but, as with all families, there is always one with a big mouth. In my case it was my dad. Bless him, he thought I'd already told her.

Finding out from someone else was worse. I was upset that I didn't get to tell her. I didn't want her to think that I was ashamed. So, when I finally saw her, she gave me that disapproving look, where she had no need to say what she thought. It was pretty obvious she was angry. She carried on with the disapproving look for a couple of weeks. Then I found out that she had

TELL ME A SECRET

told all her bridge/bingo friends, so I figured she couldn't have been that upset!

A month later she explained that it's not what she'd hoped I'd do in life, but understood that things are very different now from when she was my age. Finally, she was OK with it, but not exactly happy. I'm fine with that, because, when I'm rich, I have promised to buy her a luxury bungalow in Ireland!

I guess my family's reaction is no different to how I would react if I had kids myself.

What's your funniest moment?

My funniest moment in modelling was probably my first artistic nude shoot, which was done at famous ruins in Farnborough. I was working with a photographer, called Laurence J Power, who does mainly art shoots. He also uses one of the really old-style cameras that take ages to take the picture!

It was 6am; we met at Epsom station. It was a freezing cold morning in October, very wet and cold. We drove to Farnborough, where he set up his equipment and I got ready to bare all at the shoot. The ruins were very muddy and old. For the first pose I was in an archway of this ruin, butt-naked, freezing with muddy feet!

It was about 7.30am and the shoot was going

well. We moved to a different section of the ruin for more shots. As I picked up my stuff and ran across this muddy field butt-naked, I slipped in mud. When I looked up, there was a family of dog walkers coming towards me! So I'm stuck in mud, trying to compose myself as much as possible. The family were trying their best not to crack up laughing, but I could see they wanted to! Bless them! They literally saw everything! After that, thankfully, it started raining and so finished a very embarrassing and cold shoot.

That has to be my funniest moment in my career so far and I'm sure it will take some beating to be replaced!

What's your scariest moment?

I'd have to say my most scary moment so far had to be the Rolanda Fashion Show at the Hilton Hotel, when I was younger. This was my first-ever fashion show and I didn't have a clue what to expect. The place was full of celebrities, photographers and journalists. Basically everyone in the industry was there.

I was the most inexperienced model there, as well as the smallest too, at 5ft 6 inches. The other models were at least 5ft 8 inches, plus. I remember the moment I saw the dress I was wearing, it was very long, past my ankles and came with a massive hat that covered my face. The shoes I had with me were shoes I had had for a year or so and had been clubbed in a bit too much and the heel was wonky! I remember being extremely nervous and scared that I'd fall over in front of everyone. The other models relaxed me and showed me a few ways to walk without tripping over my dress. Finally I was ready to do it and strutted down the stage like a pro! That is definitely my scariest moment so far. But, at the same time, it gave me the confidence I have today.

Have you ever turned down work and why?

Yes, I have turned work down. I had a chance to have a fashion contract, worth a lot of money and opportunities. The person making the offer was very suggestive and tried their best to make me see this was the reality of the industry. I admittedly considered it for a week. Then came to my senses and realised that I didn't want to be successful if I had to sleep my way there. I'd never be the same person I am now if I had slept with him for a fashion contract. I may have had the career, but my quality of life wouldn't have been the same. It would have damaged me psychologically for life. So here I am starting out again, but in glamour this time. And to the person who offered me that contract, just watch me prove you wrong. It's not the way it works in the industry, because I will be successful and I will do it with my head held high, without one single sexual transaction taking place.

Do you have a sexual fantasy?
I'd have to say my sexual fantasy would be having two Vin Diesels next to me sitting in a Jacuzzi full of bubbles. Then having sex all night long on a dinner table. The whole evening would consist of lots of whipped cream, strawberries and chocolate! And yes I would love to live that fantasy!

What's your most memorable sexual encounter?
The most memorable sexual encounter I can recall took place on the M25. It was with an ex of mine called Mostak, who was Asian. We had driven to Suffolk and were on our way back from a five-hour journey. It all started by me fulfilling a certain fantasy he'd had since he was young. Of course, what man doesn't fantasise about having head while driving! So, three minutes into it, he suddenly pulls over on to the hard shoulder and we were at it like rabbits for a good hour afterwards. Many cars got a good view of my backside!

What do you think about group sex? Have you tried it?

My thoughts on group sex are that if that's what does it for you then good luck to you and go for it. I've seen it in porn films and friends of mine have tried it and loved it. Personally that's not what I'm into. Although I would happily have a threesome, any more than three would be a little too much for my liking and I imagine it would get a little bit too messy. But I'd never say 'never'. Maybe when I'm older and settled down I might want to do it then to maybe spice up the bedroom activities.

What advice would you give to someone who wanted to get into this business?

My advice would be do your research properly before deciding anything. Never take anyone's word for gospel, because this industry comes with ups and downs and many people promise things that never actually happen. Also bear in mind that this industry is run by men, so at some point in your career (more in fashion then glamour) some joker will promise you the world, contracts and all sorts if you sleep with them. This is very common and, as a model, you have to except to get a fair few offers. These people are abusing their position in this industry.

If you go down what you think is an easy route, sleeping your way into jobs, you will never know if you succeeded because you were good enough and deserve it, or because you slept your way there. Never compromise your own mental happiness for anyone or anything and also never do anything you're not 100% happy with. That's advice coming from a model that'd be in New York now if I'd not had the people around me to help me see sense.

That's my advice to all models. If you're meant to be in this industry you will be at some point. Just do it the right way.

Which bloke do you fancy the most?
Vin Diesel

Tell me a secret ... What I'm about to share with you is very hard for me and I have only shared it with a few of my very close friends.

I have always preached about doing things morally, but there was once a time that I was forced into doing something, which I now regret. It started when I got my first credit card. Being young and stupid, I decided to go on a massive shopping spree. I didn't need anything in particular; I was just living the high life, fancy restaurants and basically just wasting money. I was having fun. It was a great feeling going out and buying anything that took your fancy. Not having to look at prices on a menu, ordering the best of everything. It's really strange, but it didn't feel like I was spending money. After all no cash was dished out, just a little piece of plastic.

The crunch came when the statements started coming in. I had to make some big money and super quick time. The only thing I could think of was to go lap dancing at Sophisticats. I'd heard that you could earn a lot of money that way.

I knew that dancing alone would not clear my debts, so I put my portfolio on loads of internet modelling sites to get more shoots. I started at Sophisticats. The first night went OK. I think I made about £200, which to me wasn't bad, considering I'd never danced before and hadn't a clue what to do!

The next few nights, I clicked on to the fact that there was always twice or even three times the amount of dancers to men. So in order to make big money, you had to be really pushy which I found a little desperate and decided it wasn't for me. I also started to get a few shoots offered to me.

One assignment was for a girl/girl fetish shoot, involving cream on our feet! It was all very strange, but they were offering £350 each. I asked a friend who is also a model and we went to Lancashire for the shoot. When we turned up, it was clear that a lot of people are apparently into feet fetishes, so we thought, Why not?

Although this was not a way I wanted to progress my career, we were desperate and needed the cash at the time, but eventually made the most of it and saw the funny side in the job. We had a good laugh. It was so stupid that it was hilariously funny. I made good money and, shortly after, got myself out of trouble financially. My friend and I still look back at that shoot and laugh. My mate even has a copy of the picture, which she decided to put up in her kitchen!

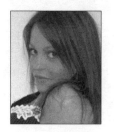

ZOE DEE

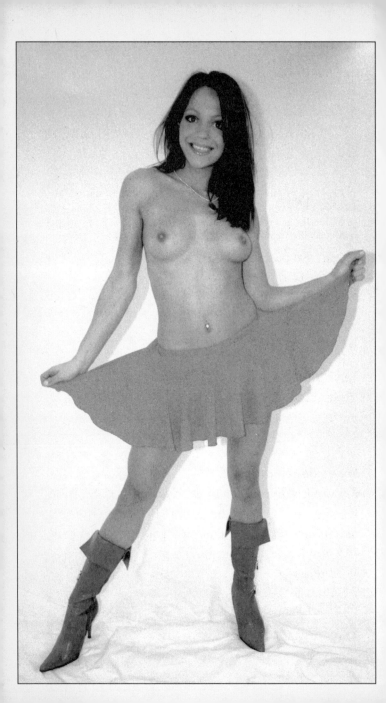

ZOE DEE

Name: Pippa Lee
Model/Dance Name: Zoe Dee
Star Sign: Scorpio
Age: 19
Vital Stats: 32C-22-32
Lives: West Midlands
Fave Food: Italian and Chinese
Fave Drink: Bailey's Latte

Where do you work?

I currently live close to the National Exhibition Centre in Birmingham so I get a lot of assignments to model and do promo work at a lot of shows and exhibitions there. I usually get at least one job a month at the NEC.

I do a lot of modelling work locally to where I live, but I also have jobs that take me around the UK. I like to travel and see new places. It's great experience for me when my modelling takes me further afield. Funnily enough, I had never been on a plane or even outside of England until I was 18 so you can imagine how excited I was when, last year, I did the Dublin Motorbike Show. It was my first flight and my first assignment out of the country. If anyone was on the same flight, I was the one who didn't stop smiling the whole flight.

Last year was a good year for work outside of the UK. I got another job in Dublin and I also got to work at an exhibition in Brno, in the Czech Republic. I was working for an English company and was working with another model. We had a great time over in the Czech Republic. There were some fantastic restaurants and beautiful architecture. I'd love to go back there to visit some day.

How did you get into modelling?

I wanted to be a model and a dancer when I was a little girl – isn't it every little girl's dream? When I was about nine, I turned into a bit of a tomboy and developed a huge phobia of cameras. I absolutely hated anyone taking pictures of me. Gradually my dreams of being a model disappeared and my confidence faded.

One day on my way to work, while reading a local newspaper, the *Metro*, I spotted an advert for auditions that were being held at an out-of-town table dancing club, Club Arcadia, in West Brom. It promised high pay, free training and friendly environment. I hated my job in retail, so it really got me to think. I tore out the advert and put it in my bag. All day at work it was really playing on my mind. So much so that as soon as I got home I called the number and arranged an audition for the next evening.

I went along and passed the audition. Since then I have just tried to move on and up. Getting into this line of work has made me feel complete. It's great doing a job that I like and that I'm good at.

What's the biggest fee/tip you have ever earned?

My biggest fee was probably for a catalogue and calendar that I shot. It was done in the South East and it took a few days to shoot. I had a great time. I can't tell you how much I got paid because of discretion to the client, but I will say I was looked after really well. Treated like a princess. It was lovely.

What famous people have you danced and modelled for? What highstreet publications have you been in?

I went for my first screen test a short while ago. It was for a presenting job on Television X. The producer got me to read from a script to camera. It was a bit daunting but I was told I did well and by the time you are reading this I will probably be on the channel.

I have also done a few bits and pieces for *Nuts* magazine. I love modelling for *Nuts* – I have such a laugh. The guys from the magazine are great fun and really know how to have a good time.

What other work have you done?

I had my first job when I was about 14. I was a kitchen assistant in an old people's home called the Babalake House, in Meriden. I didn't really like it because it meant that I was stuck in a kitchen instead of being out with my friends having fun. Five days a week I would head down to the old people's home to do my two-hour shift. I hated it.

Eventually I parted company with the oldies and went into waiting on tables and housekeeping at a local hotel, The Windmill Village in Coventry. Eventually I also got bored of this and left.

After I left the hotel I started as a shopfloor assistant at T J Hughes, in Coventry, in the ladies- and childrenswear section. I really enjoyed it; I found it very easy and got on with the people I worked with really well. I must have impressed somebody because within about a month I was called into the manager's office and promoted to a supervisor position. I was 17 by this time and getting promoted for the first time gave me a little confidence boost.

My role as a supervisor was to make sure the stock was put out on time, cash up and make sure all the staff were working. It was a big role for me to have at such a young age, but I really enjoyed it.

When I was in control of the floor staff, they worked their bollocks off. But after a few months new management came in and started to change a lot of this. Staff were coming and going all the time and I started to not want to be there any more. Maybe it was fate making me move on, because if I had been happy I probably wouldn't have applied for the audition for the table dancers.

When I first started modelling it was really hard because I was totally new to it all. I was a very small fish in a very big pond. I had been brought up to be pretty streetwise and to know a good card from a bad one. All the dodgy photographers, porn producers and weirdos love new models. These guys know that they stand a good chance with a new model, because she doesn't know anyone in the industry. All they know is that these girls are still very naïve about the industry and desperate to make it as a model. I had all kinds of strange offers when I first started modelling and still do. You can spot the dodgy ones; they always have very weird requests. But I have also had some really bizarre ones in; here's an example of one I received recently:

> Hey, I love your work very much. I saw you on a website.
>
> I am an 18 year old girl. I want to become a model like you but I am 6'11"(210cm tall, 7'6"(228cm) in my highest heels. I wanna do photoshoots with other women. But nobody wants to stand next to me.
> Now my questions to you:
> - HOW TALL ARE YOU? ARE YOU ALSO TALL OR NOT?
> - WOULD YOU DO A PHOTOSHOOT WITH A GIRL AS TALL AS ME IF YOU KNOW YOU WOULD ONLY COME UP TO HER CHEST IF YOU WEAR YOUR SUPERHIGH HEELS?
> - HOW TALL WAS THE TALLEST WOMAN YOU HAVE STAND NEXT TO OR WORKED WITH?
> - TILL WHERE DID YOU COME, HER SHOULDER OR WHERE?

ZOE DEE

PLEASE ANSWER THESE THREE QUESTIONS. IT WOULD BE A GREAT SUPPORT TO ME.

THANKS

Guess they don't come stranger than that one.

I have worked hard to get with a lot of agencies, in order that I can get enough assignments for modelling to be my full-time career. I normally work six days a week, whether it be on shoots, at shows, working on my website or answering emails. I like to keep myself busy. I think I would find it hard to go back to a 9–5 Mon–Fri career. Don't get me wrong, being a model isn't easy. There are a lot of long hours, late nights and early mornings. You also have to have pretty thick skin because there are some nasty criticising people with really big opinions out there – they make Simon Cowell look like a piece of wet lettuce. I love it and I consider myself really lucky to be doing something I love so much.

Do you have any famous friends?

Manchester comedian Mike McLean is a fan of mine. It's strange because when I was young I wrote to him and asked him for his autograph. The other month I got an email from him asking me for mine.

TELL ME A SECRET

What does your family think of the work you do?

My mum thought I was joking when I told her that I wanted to get into pole dancing, especially when I told her that I had replied to an ad in a newspaper. I have had a lot of fads in my life and I suppose she thought it was just another one.

My dad wasn't really bothered by it; he didn't dislike me doing it, although he did take the mickey a bit at first.

My family has always been really laidback about it all. I got a lot better at dancing and, after I won a lap-dancing award, my family really did make it known to me how proud they all were. Before I started dancing I can't remember a time when I had made my parents proud. I guess that's really sad.

When I started modelling they were even happier, especially my dad, he was so proud of me. When I was growing up I was a real daddy's girl. I used to go everywhere with him, including the pub. When I had my first appearance in the paper, he took it in his local pub and showed it to all his friends. The funny thing was I was topless in the paper. That's how proud he was. He didn't care what I was doing as long as I was happy and doing it well.

Unfortunately I lost my dad in late September 2004. He was 61 and died of emphysema. He passed away peacefully in his sleep, and it was unexpected, so I didn't get to say goodbye to him. It helps knowing how proud he was of me, seeing his face, full of pride, when he smiled at me.

I'm fortunate because I now have a really close relationship with my mum and sister; they are two of my closest friends, which, once upon a time, I thought would be impossible. I wasn't the easiest of children and must have caused them a lot of grief when I was young. But now I can talk to them about anything, we all help each other whenever and however we can. I don't know what I would do without them. I get a lot of support from both my family and my boyfriend.

What's your funniest moment?

My funniest moment was probably my last birthday. It's one that I won't forget in a hurry. My boyfriend Charlie (DJ Charma) had taken me out for a really nice romantic meal in Birmingham. It was a Sunday evening so it was pretty quiet in town. After finishing the meal, it was still quite early, so we decided that we would go and see *Alfie* at the Odeon on New Street.

It wasn't a long walk to the cinema but, on the way there, we stopped at a stall at the bottom of New Street that was selling giant teddies. They are not normally my 'thing', but I fell in love with a 4 ft Tigger and asked my boyfriend to buy it for me. He was a bit dubious because it was so big and we were on our way to the cinema. It was my birthday and I wasn't going to take no for an answer so, bless him, he bought it for me.

There we were staggering off in the centre of Birmingham with our new companion, a 4 ft Tigger. My boyfriend refused to carry him, because he was scared of looking feminine, so I had to carry it. I was wearing heels, which didn't make it easy. But to my amazement we finally got to the cinema. When we got to the ticket office they tried to charge us extra, as they said that Tigger would take up a seat of his own. After a bit of persuasion and a few comments such as, 'Are you taking the piss?', we managed to laugh it off with the person behind the till and made our way to our seats.

We sat down, Tigger with a seat of his own and watched the film. Just as we were coming out of our screen, someone tapped me on the shoulder. 'Are you Zoe? I'm such a big fan.' I was mortified. Of all the times to be spotted by a fan was the time when I'm accompanied by an overgrown teddy bear. To make it worse he had a camera and insisted that he wanted a picture of me and Tigger. How could I refuse? So I smiled sweetly and posed with my furry friend, even though inside I was cringing with embarrassment. I'd love to see the picture; I bet my face was bright red. It always makes me giggle when I think about it.

What's your scariest moment?

My scariest moment was definitely going for my first audition to be a pole dancer. I had applied at a small out-of-town club; I applied on a Thursday and was asked to go in the next evening for an audition. For some silly reason I agreed that that would be fine. I don't know why because I normally like to give myself time to prepare for things. But I kind of felt that if I didn't go to the club next day I'd bottle out and never go through with it again. I didn't want to go to Spearmint Rhino or Legs 11 for my first audition because they are big clubs with a lot of professional, talented girls working there. I didn't know whether I would be able to do it. I could barely dance, let alone dance around a pole.

The next day I spent all day getting myself ready. While tanning, preening and plucking, I got myself really worked up. I was so nervous. Eventually the evening came around; I packed some make-up and a little black dress in a bag and set out for the club. I was very nervous. I thought that I would be auditioning before the

TELL ME A SECRET

club opened and before the other girls arrived, so this was putting my mind at rest slightly.

I got to the club, but it was still closed. There were a few dancers waiting outside to be let in, which was the last thing I wanted. I didn't want to see anyone in case I messed up the audition. If no one saw me then it didn't matter as much and I could just pretend that it had never happened.

The doors eventually opened. As soon as I was let in, they asked me to get changed and then they would tell me more about the audition.

The changing room was so small and cramped; I don't think I have ever seen so many girls getting changed and trying to put make-up on in such a small place. It felt a bit like a cattle market. I felt really insignificant amongst all the other dancers. I was still very young, small and inexperienced. I put on my make-up and little black dress as quickly as I could and went to find the manager. I just wanted to get my audition over and done with as soon as possible.

By the time he appeared, most of the girls were dressed and ready for work. He asked me what I wanted to drink and took me over to one of the tables in front of the pole. We had a chat and he told me what the job involved. No problems so far. Then he dropped it on me. 'So now all you have to do it get up on that pole and show me what you can do.' He looked at me and smiled.

'What, now?' I shrieked.

'Of course,' he said, like I should have known better.

So I took a deep breath and made my way up on to the stage.

Once I was up there I could see the whole club. I could see at least a dozen girls making themselves comfortable at tables around the room, ready to watch me at my scariest moment. I could see the manager looking up at me, waiting for my performance. I bet he loved watching girls on the pole for the first time, I thought. I took a deep breath and just went for it. I must have done something right, because the manager liked me. He said that he would love to have me work at the club. So the following evening I started working at the club.

As time passed my skills on the pole improved and so did my confidence. I learned by watching the other girls and then combining their moves with some of my own techniques. I stayed at the club until I felt I was ready to move on to bigger things. I am really proud of myself having the balls to go to such a pressured audition. Now I don't really get scared or nervous, I just enjoy it.

Have you ever turned down work and why?
I am very selective about the work I take on.

TELL ME A SECRET

There are so many scams, degrading assignments and weirdos out there. When taking on an assignment you not only have to think about whether you're going to be comfortable doing it, but also whether it is going to be good for your career and good promotion for yourself. You are your work.

I used to get a lot of emails from the *Trisha* show's office asking me if I have anything I'd like to talk about on the show or if I would like to appear in one of the many episodes featuring models. I would rather be in the audience watching *Trisha* than be on stage washing my dirty lingerie in public.

Then there was *Babe Station/Cast*, no offence to the models on the show, because I know a few, but I could never do that. For those of you who haven't seen *Babe Station/Cast*, it is models in a studio talking to people on the phone on a live TV show, flashing, reading text messages and doing as they are asked by the people on the phone. Really low budget and it has a terrible reputation for being tasteless. One model was once meant to have said, excuse me for saying this but it is a quote, 'I'm as happy as a paedophile in a playground.' I wouldn't do it for all the money in the world.

When I started modelling, I knew exactly

where I wanted to go with my modelling and what standards I would go to. There are many temptations and many offers; like in the beginning of my modelling career I got approached by lots of porn makers, dodgy photographers and websites. They were all hoping to get a naïve model with no direction, just so they can lead her down the wrong path. I didn't, and still don't, even respond when I get offers of work out of my boundaries.

Do you have a sexual fantasy?
I hate to fulfil fantasies because once a fantasy has been fulfilled it is no longer a fantasy, but a memory. So if it is to be fulfilled it has got to be just perfect.

My fantasy that I have not fulfilled, yet, is jetting off to a Caribbean island with the man I love. We stay in an exquisite hotel in an exotic location. After dining at a beautiful restaurant, we drink expensive Champagne, listen to romantic music. Then hand in hand we go for a walk along on a deserted moonlit beach. We stop and sit down close to the bottom of the cliffs to listen to the waves and look at the stars. My man starts to kiss my neck as we gradually lie down on the sand … You can imagine what happens next.

It's inevitable that I will fulfil my fantasy some day, but when, I don't know.

What's your most memorable sexual experience?

My boyfriend and I have a special place, which isn't very far from where we live. This place is really special because, not long after we had first met, he was walking me home one night and this is where my boyfriend and me had our first kiss and cuddle. It's like a secret garden; it's so remote. In the summer it is pretty with wild flowers and big oak trees to sit under. So whenever it is a nice summer's day and we get bored we go to our secret garden and relive our first intimate moments.

What do you think about group sex? Have you tried it?

I have never tried it, never fantasised about it, or even thought about doing it. In fact the thought of group sex scares me slightly. I knew a few dancers once that were into that kind of thing. They used to go to swingers' parties and adult fetish parties – you name it they were up for the lot and they loved it. Different strokes for different folks, I suppose. Personally, the thought of bits and pieces of naked bodies everywhere alarms me a bit. I wouldn't know where to put myself.

What advice would you give someone who wanted to get into this business?

I'd advise anyone who wants to get into modelling to research the industry as much as they can before they even go for their first shoot or join with their first agency. You have to be so careful because there are many people out there waiting to rip you off in this industry. You should only work for people that you have heard good reports about. There are agencies and photographers that will promise you the world, fame, fortune, glamour, anything you want. But be warned, if the offer sounds too good to be true, then it probably is.

Modelling isn't an easy thing to get into. Your look has to be right for the market, or the particular market you are trying to break into. Don't let me put you off trying because there are agencies out there which do look after your needs, but not all of them. That's why it's good to go with a recommendation. There are plenty of agencies out there – you just have to find one that suits you and your look.

The most important things are to keep your confidence, a strong will and most of all, be careful. When I have a daughter, if she is anything like me, then of course I'd let her model. I'd support her and help her as much as she wanted me to.

TELL ME A SECRET

Which bloke do you fancy the most?
Mine of course!

Tell me a secret ... I do a lot of my lingerie and topless modelling work, obviously, because of the size of my boobs and I work hard to keep my body in shape but it hasn't always been this way.

I have always been quite short (5' 3"), which I don't mind, I like being small but I think this is why I didn't develop any boobs at all, until I was 16. This was a big problem to me growing up; a lot of girls in my year at school had huge boobs and I was so jealous. All the boys were permanently talking about them, saying how great they were.

I use to spend ages looking at myself in the mirror, hating what I saw. Enough was enough. One day when getting ready to go to school I had an idea, I reached for the cotton wool and applied an even layer inside each cup of my bra. I knew I could only put a little in otherwise it would have been blatantly obvious. But I made my boobs about a size bigger. What I failed to think about at the time, was that I would now have to maintain padding my bra until I grew boobs, had a boob job or left school. I never told anyone about this and never had – until now that is.

PE was a nightmare because we had a

perverted PE teacher, who liked to see the girls in the shower naked, and, of course, we had to take our bras and knickers off before showering after PE, which, when you are young, it's embarrassing enough having to share a shower, let alone having to try and take off a stuffed bra without anyone noticing and having a shower without anyone seeing how big my boobs were.

In the end I used to just tell the teachers I had an injury to get out of doing PE. Then I wouldn't have to have a shower, problem solved. I later moved schools to do my exams and I'm glad I did because I was getting through so much cotton wool it was untrue. I have to laugh about it now. I often imagine how many conversations guys had about my cotton wool boobs – if only they knew.

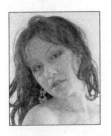

YVETTE

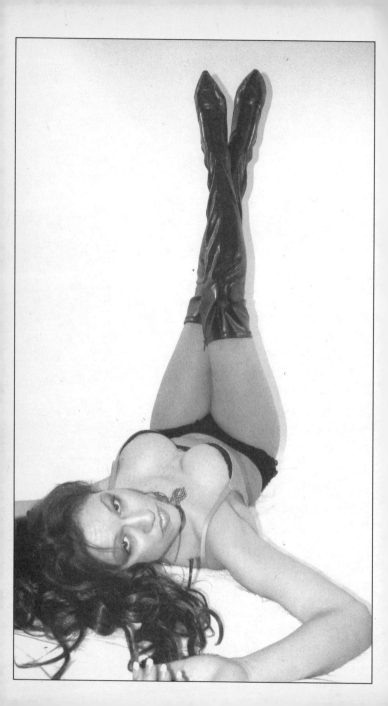

YVETTE

Name: Yvette Michelle Merriman
Dance Name: Briony
Model name: Yvette
Star Sign: Taurus
Age: 21
Vital Stats: 32D-25-35
Lives: Surrey
Fave Food: Mexican
Fave Drink: I'm a complete lightweight so I love wine, but normally abstain – 'cause I get naughty when I'm drunk!

Where do you work?

I use to work at Spearmint Rhino's Gentleman's Club – Tottenham Court Road and Colnbrook. I am also with three glamour-modelling agencies at the moment – Models-inc.co.uk, Zoommodels.co.uk and vipmodels.co.uk. I do photographic work (including nude shots but only showing breasts totally exposed). I also work at car shows as a promo girl – I have done events such as *Max Power*, Hot Import Nights Car Show at Earl's Court and I came third out of 20-plus girls for the title of Miss HIN 2004.

It was only recently that I stopped working at Spearmint Rhino. I was based out at the Colnbrook Spearmint Rhino, but also danced at the Tottenham Court Road (TCR), mainly over the Christmas period. The money is much better with the tourists in London. The main difference is that Colnbrook is mainly filled with businessmen that are staying in hotels around the Heathrow area and London is tourists and office parties of guys that are curious about lap-dancing clubs and don't pay any money!!!

Colnbrook club is also filled with married men – don't ever trust your husband if they say they are going to London on 'business', 'cause the first thing they do is ask, 'where's the nearest lap-dancing club'. I can also tell you that majority of them ask the girls if they do 'extras'.

The regular girls get tipped off by the bouncers as to who has chips – or loads of cash – and points them in the right direction. When guys come to the club for the first time, they always ask the bouncers who should dance for them – whatever girl is sleeping or sucking that bouncer that week gets the cash-rich punters.

YVETTE

If you have a bouncer on your side you can earn a lot of money. Naturally, if the bouncer gets the girl money, she also sorts him out with a tip for his trouble – cash or kindness!

London is the place to be to dance for famous people – to be fair when I first started I was so young and naive that I didn't recognise anyone. I just kept my head down and danced. The more experienced girls get the famous guys with the money. Now I've been out and about on the London party scene, I would catch everyone out straight away …

How did you get into modelling?

My mother was always entering me into modelling competitions from a young age and I did pretty OK at it. I managed to get through to the Elite Look of the Year for quite a few years running – but I wasn't considered quirky enough. I never really understood what that meant! The idea of modelling just naturally carried on through my teens.

I grew up in Las Vegas, which meant I did not want a normal 9–5 job. But my mum passed away when I was 15, which meant I really didn't have any other choice but to join the rat race. The modelling thing has always been at the back of my mind but I didn't think I was pretty enough to really cut it.

I started modelling with local amateur

photographers when I was 20. I managed to really get my big break about a year after that, when I went to the *Max Power* Car Show in Birmingham and got 'spotted' by a couple of agencies.

In February 2002 I had a really bad car accident. I spent over a year recovering. I never thought that I would ever be a lap dancer. But I had medical and dental bills that needed paying and I only earned around £15K a year in my day job. A friend of mine, who had been doing it for years, got me an audition and I got taken on straight away in November 2003. I paid off my bills and managed to pay a deposit on a new car too.

What's the biggest fee/tip you have ever earned?

Biggest tip was well over £1,000 – but I got paid in Rhino chips so after commission I ended up taking home £800. 'Rhino chips' are a way for the guys to pay for dances if they haven't got cash. They can have their card charged for the amount of dances they want to have – in return they get chips that look like casino chips, with a picture of a girl on the front and back. You can get £10 chips and £20 chips. Topless dances are £10 and the fully nude dances are £20. The girls don't like getting paid in chips in London as the club takes a massive commission off the top – normally around £7 out of every £20.

YVETTE

I don't know what I did to deserve the £1,000. It was a group of Arabs who had hired a private room for the night; they paid the doormen to find them girls and we were expected to stay with them the whole night.

What famous people have you danced or modelled for?

The most famous people I have danced for to date are the Chelsea Football Club and David Blaine. According to the girls that were working with me that night, CFC go there all the time. And now I've got to know the guys a bit better it does seem to be true. Their training ground used to be in Heathrow, so they would always go to the club at Colnbrook, but their ground has now moved to Cobham so no one has seen them for a while. (Well, not at Colnbrook anyway!!)

I remember one time when I danced for them. They were all out for John Terry's birthday (8.12.03) – I did a few lap dances for the team and exchanged numbers with a player or two! I was fairly liberal with giving my number out to anyone. I was single and, actually, I did meet some genuinely nice, fun guys through the club.

I have kept in touch with a few of the players since I first danced for them and have made a few friendships on the team. I get invited to their

Christmas parties and more recently the PFA do that was held in London, as well as the after-party at Elysium nightclub. Guess I must have given Wayne Bridge one hell of a dance! He, he!!!!

Although I did get myself in a bit of a tricky situation with one of the players one night. Wayne Bridge's cousin invited me back to Wayne's house after a party. Wayne was crashed out upstairs and I was just chatting to the cousin.

As we were chatting Wayne's girlfriend came back to the house. She was well pissed off when she saw me there but I think I convinced her that nothing had gone on with Wayne. He had gone straight to bed when we got back. However, it wasn't that simple, because the next day the girlfriend got hold of my mobile number, which was on Wayne's telephone. His cousin had used his phone to call me but she obviously thought he had been ringing me. She rang me and asked if I was the same girl that was at the house the evening before and I told her I was. She hung up even more pissed off. The funny thing was that Wayne rang me about half-an-hour later. He was pretty shocked when he heard she had called. Not sure what happened between them but they're still together so obviously it got sorted.

YVETTE

What other work have you done?

Like the majority of people I've worked in cafés and bars in the past for extra money.

Modelling is a part-time career/hobby. I haven't really had a chance to dedicate myself to it 100 per cent. I had been waiting to have a breast augmentation to help my career, which I finally had done on 30/09/04 (momentous date and intend to celebrate it like my birthday – well, after all, something was created and born!). Therefore, I developed from a 32A/B to a proud and firm 32D.

Aside from my regular dance work in the clubs, I also work on boat parties with other lap dancers. You can earn a lot more money away from the clubs and the extortionate commission they charge us!

Now the boring part – my day job! Well, actually I have just jacked my job, as my modelling assignments were covering enough to live on. So up until recently I was an investment analyst at an actuarial firm (yawn, yawn, and yes, I know, almost as bad as saying I'm an accountant).

Do you have any famous friends?

I know the Chelsea squad on a first-name basis and get invited on nights out with the players. Also I can count Frank Sinclair and Marcus Bent as friends – although their other halves might be surprised to learn that! (PS I haven't slept with any of these guys – we are *just* friends!) Also by going to watch Chelsea play I've got to know some of the players' families like Scott Parker's brother. And I've seen some of the *EastEnders* cast up there on a regular basis.

What does your family think of the work you do?

I am lucky in that I am very close to my 'adopted family'. It took me a little while to really settle in and get used to the family unit – i.e. having a mum and a dad always around and having brothers and sisters for the first time. At the moment my sister is my manager. She does all my administrative work and gets me the majority of my bookings. We are lucky that we have a very good working relationship. I'm godmother to her daughter and we are close inside and outside of our working relationship.

My family doesn't know I work as a lap dancer. If they ever suspected they would not be happy. My adoptive parents are not as liberal as my birth parents (my mum was a showgirl in Vegas – she got her boobs out every night for half the money I earn!). But I'm old enough to do what I want, I guess – and, if they did find out through this book, then I wouldn't really care about their reaction. They are positive about the modelling because they know I struggle on my wages and they know that I want more than ever to move out and be more independent. They like my sister being my manager, because it means that eventually she won't have to work in an office either.

It's not like they are prudes or anything. They were very happy for me when I said I wanted to get my boobs done – they were fascinated to see the results!!

What's your funniest moment?

It has to be Christmas 2003. We were allowed to wear anything we wanted at Spearmint as long as it had a Christmas theme – I spent all my nights running around as a Mrs Claus and had the best time ever. The only problem was dancing on the bar topless. My Santa hat fell off; I slipped on it and fell in to the bar, the drinks and the customers. In my shoes I'm over 6'2" – and they were not happy with me. It happened more than once. Needless to say, I was not the most graceful of lap dancers. I was always getting told off for falling over mid-dance into customers' laps and landing right on their little erections. Although I don't think the clients were bothered, as I always got the biggest tips from the guys I fell on!

TELL ME A SECRET

What's your scariest moment?

David Blaine came in after his famous 'box over the River Thames' stunt. He was with his girlfriend and they took a booth near the back of the club. He was surrounded by dancers and his girlfriend was being a lot more friendly and talkative to them than he was.

I spoke to David briefly – but his girlfriend seemed to be flirting with me. Her behaviour certainly struck me as a bit weird. Both of them were really disturbing in that you couldn't look at them in the eyes without it freaking you out. Their eyes were very hypnotic and piercing. I felt that he could almost read my mind just by looking at me.

I used to get lots of general scary moments most nights – when you have to dance for the guys that get sexually excited and turned on by your dancing and they call you filthy names. I've been called some horrible stuff and been told what some guys would like to do to me given half the chance. It's disgusting. There is a general club rule that under no circumstances are you allowed to touch the dancer. However, you can't do a thing about people being perverted and gobby. You just have to blank them out.

Have you ever turned down work and why?

I have turned down the offer of appearing on

YVETTE

Babe/Cast on a regular basis because my parents were getting a bit prudish about me wiggling around on a bed for three hours on live TV touching myself up and talking dirty on the phone. I had a laugh but there are certain feelings I have to consider while living in their house.

Also I have had to regularly turn down offers of going back to hotel rooms to be paid for sex/sexual acts. The other part of the job (and some would say perk) is when doing a dance the guy offers you more money if you will touch him or vice versa. They don't understand that there are cameras in the club and that they are being watched. The money is tempting, but I have watched girls let guys stick their fingers up them just for an extra £5. It's very degrading.

Do you have a sexual fantasy?
It would be to have sex with a really fit guy, with a couple of girls either watching or joining in, or maybe both!

What's your most memorable sexual encounter?
It was in Greece. I was with my boyfriend at the time. It was hot and we were making love on the beach. It was quick, passionate and very memorable.

TELL ME A SECRET

**What do you think about group sex?
Have you tried it?**
If that is what people are in to then that's great. It's not something I would really take part in – but I wouldn't mind watching.

What advice would you give someone who wanted to get into this business?
Get someone older, or in your family, to help you and look out for you. There are so many people out there ready to rip you off!

Which bloke do you fancy the most?
A mixture between Mathew McConaughey and Vin Diesel.

Tell me a secret ... I guess my biggest secret is *me*! People I know and people I have met in the past think of me as a strong character. A woman who knows what she wants and who is full of confidence. Truth is, I'm not. I battle every day with trusting people. I think this lack of trust in people has made me a hard person where feelings and emotions are concerned.

I never talk about my past with anyone because it is good for me to hide behind this confident character. I have always thought that, if I tell people about myself, it would make me

YVETTE

vulnerable. An easy target to hurt. I was sexually abused as a child, but now I think I am strong enough to talk about who I really am.

I didn't have the most stable of upbringings. I have not seen my father since I was a child. For all I know he could be dead by now.

My mum was a showgirl in Vegas – originally born in Surrey, England. She went out there when she was 22. To my knowledge, we have mirrored each other in regards to luck with men. She was married twice – the first to a casino owner's son, Fred Morledge, that she loved with all her heart. But they eventually called it a day due to complications.

After that (quite a few years later) she met my father, Robert Bishop. He was an insurance salesman – and I don't know much more. When my mum found out she was dying of cancer she tried to tell me as much as she could about her life. Naturally this wasn't the entire truth as I was still only 15 and, although she had stuff to tell me, I don't think she wanted me to have too much to deal with. It was always a touchy subject talking about my dad. Regardless of what happened to me, I still wanted to know my history and where I came from.

After my mum died I found the marriage certificate. It turned out that my parents only married two months before I was born. Hardly the story of love and being conceived by a husband and wife like I had been told. I then thought, What else had my mother said to me that wasn't the whole truth? I may never know.

I came to England when I was 10. My mum died when I was 15 and I was then placed with the family I live with now.

At 16 I was still a virgin and had planned to be until I met my future husband. My mum had been hurt enough by lots of guys and I was adamant it wasn't going to happen to me. I had been brought up in such a strict religious household, where it was unheard of to be having sex – especially before the age of 18.

My mum was liberal in that we could talk about anything, but I was very sheltered and protected – I wasn't even allowed to have sleepovers if my mum didn't know their parents!

When I was 16 I started dating. James was a bouncer at my local nightclub. I was a bit naïve and I only liked going out with him 'cause I used to get in for free! We never even snogged – he was a massive black guy about 6'5" and built like a brick shithouse. I think it was the fact that I thought he could protect me. I'm not really sure why I was attracted to him. We seemed such a mish-mash couple. He even came to my house and met my adoptive parents.

YVETTE

It was New Year's Eve and I was in the club James worked in. I never drank alcohol and did not realize that my orange juice had been spiked.

I started to feel quite ill. James was not concerned. He took me round the back of the club and had sex with me. Then he put me in a cab home, incoherent and covered in blood.

I woke the next morning not knowing why I was covered in blood. I just thought I had come on my period. But when I got out of bed I knew what had happened. The horrors of the night before came flooding back. I could hardly walk with the pain inside me. I was torn between having a bath and getting over it and freaking out if he had used protection or not. I didn't tell anyone.

After this happened, James disappeared and his mobile number changed. I saw him a few months later with a girl. He just smiled at me and said 'hi' like there was nothing wrong. I was too shocked with the fact I had even seen him to say a word. I just ran away.

From then on I didn't feel special or pure and vowed to never let anyone hurt me like that again. He took something physical but he never knew my mind and never got to know who I really am. So he missed out on a great girl for one sordid night.

I hope that this isn't true – but he may well have ruined my trust in men for the rest of my life. It is going to take one hell of a special guy to earn my undying love and trust.

I'm not sure whether I started dancing because it gave me power over the men. But it made me feel good having this power. The only problem was that the whole time I was dancing I could never really take it seriously. There were the money-hungry girls that were constantly on the look-out for a sugar daddy that would pay for their new boobs or their hair extensions. But I am so independent I just couldn't sit there and talk crap with sad old guys on the off-chance they might throw me some extra money.

Maybe that was my downfall as to why I didn't ever get really really successful. The more successful girls had regulars. These are guys that come just to see one girl and won't go for dances or talk to anyone else. I don't know what went/goes on with a girl and her regular ... One can only guess.

I have been offered thousands of pounds for sexual favours and keeping lonely businessmen company. The footballers and better-looking men of the world never bother to make these kinds of offers because they know they could get a girl without having to pay for it.

YVETTE

My most recent example of an offer is a guy I will call John, not his real name. He is 'happily' married to a woman many years his junior. He is a business man in the area. He was constantly telling me how much money he has and what he could buy me. He was by no means bad-looking and we very nearly did meet up. But with us both being busy people it just didn't materialise. He was offering to buy me a place to live. I nearly entered the cliché of being a kept woman by some older guy I met in a strip club. I can definitely see how girls get into these situations. You don't want to have to get naked for £20 when there's a guy offering to give you so much more.

I have never been tempted to take up offers of being paid for sex. It is something I hope I never lower myself to because you can use your shell for making money – but I never want to let someone buy my most intimate parts and places. As long as I'm healthy and can earn money other ways, I will never prostitute myself.

I have tried to strike up relationships with guys I've met at night doing my job, but it has never worked out. I did see a guy for a few months that I met while working, but it didn't go anywhere. He came in for a mate's stag do and we just got chatting. I didn't do any dances for them in the end because we had struck up a friendship and I didn't want to lose that. We met up for drinks and stuff but he just couldn't get over the fact I stripped and had to tell all his mates that he was dating a stripper. As a result. I never got any respect from him and he used me. He never would have taken me home to meet mummy and daddy. I was only ever good enough to hang off his arm to show off to his mates.

This line of work does make you a sceptic and, to be fair, I was single for nearly two years because I had been propositioned by too many 'loving fathers, husbands, fiancés and boyfriends' to make me think that any guy could be faithful and perfect. Maybe I still believe that now, that no one is truly happy with what they have at home and they will always be looking for something more – whether it's a lap dance, a porn mag or looking for a faceless slag in a club to suck their cock.

I have not met one guy in the last two-plus years that has been faithful and talked about the woman they have at home with the respect they deserve. I am searching for the simplest pleasures in life – yet they seem to be the hardest to find. I want a guy who appreciates me for who I am. Who respects that I do a hard job to pay the bills and it is *only a job*! No matter what I am doing I am emotionless – and my heart will be with my

YVETTE

guy not with the faceless stranger I am dancing for or speaking to.

As far as I am concerned I earn an honest living – just because I don't wear a lot of clothes in my job, that does not make it an invalid profession. It will take a special person to look at me and see who I am under the make-up, fake boobs and sexy clothes. All I want is a family, nice house and not have to struggle for every penny. I would love to be successful and get the fame, but I think that a family and someone who loves me would fill the void better than millions in the bank.

At the moment I have met someone that I see a future with – to say that I already love him would not be a lie. If I was still working as an investment analyst we would probably be in a church right now exchanging our vows (well almost!!). But I am having to prove myself to all his friends and family – more so than I ever thought I would. I wish there wasn't, but there is a stereotype attached to this profession and it makes all guys think they can bed you. All women are uncomfortable in your presence and all parents wish you weren't dating their son. Little do people know that we haven't even seen each other without clothes on. I feel sorry for him because I am driven to prove to him that I am a moral, nice girl and not some slapper – so the poor boy is gonna be waiting a long time for the 'Yvette love'!!

I feel that we might always have obstacles to face – but if he is half the man he appears to be then he will take the time to get to know me and we will overcome them together.

Sod's Law, I'll be single again by the time this goes to print!!